Herself

by E. B. Lowry

PREFACE

A recent number of the Journal of the American Medical Association contained this paragraph:

"A correspondent asks for a good book describing the female generative organs anatomically, physiologically and pathologically, treating also of childbirth, written in language easily understood by a layman. He desires to give copies to some of his young women patients. The editor regrets there is no satisfactory book on the subject although there is great need for one."

It is a lamentable fact that the majority of women and girls are ignorant of the structure of their most important organs. In the majority of schools and colleges where physiology is taught, absolutely nothing is mentioned about the reproductive organs. As far as books or instruction are concerned, the girl is ignorant of their very existence. If she knew something of the structure of such important organs and the harmful results of many practices or acts of carelessness affecting them, would she not be better prepared to take the proper care of herself and more liable to develop into a strong, healthy woman?

If a girl in the business world is intrusted with a delicate piece of machinery she is taught the structure, use and care of it. Why is it not just as necessary that the girl, who is intrusted with the care of delicate organisms upon whose condition depends the health of the future generation, be instructed regarding the care of these organs? Instead, she is left in absolute ignorance and then blamed if she mars them.

Every woman should have some knowledge of the structure and care of her body, especially of those parts which are concerned so intimately in the welfare of the future generation. Every woman, too, should receive some instruction regarding the care of young children and the proper management of the home. A woman who attempts to care for herself and her children without proper knowledge of these subjects is like a man who tries to run his business blindfolded.

That thinking women are awakening to the fact that they have been suffering unnecessarily and are realizing the necessity for more knowledge concerning the hygiene and physiology of their own bodies is shown by the fact that nearly every chapter in this book has been written in answer to questions asked by women readers of the author's magazine articles. With the hope that the plain facts herein set forth will aid some women to have healthier and happier lives and healthier and happier babies this series of talks has been written.

CONTENTS

CHAPTER I

ANATOMY AND PHYSIOLOGY OF THE FEMALE ORGANS

Before we can understand the care of anything we must have some knowledge of its structure; so I think it well, in this our first talk, that we should learn something of the structure of the female generative organs. As I have told some of you in former talks, the womb is designed as a nest for the babe during its process of development from the egg or ovule. It lies in the center of the pelvis, or lower part of the body cavity, in front of the rectum and behind and above the bladder. It is pear-shaped, with the small end downward, and is about three inches long, two inches wide and one inch thick. It consists of layers of muscles enclosing a cavity which, owing to the thickness of the walls, is comparatively small. This cavity is triangular in shape and has three openings,--one at the lower end or mouth of the womb into the vagina and one at each side, near the top, into the fallopian tubes. The womb, or uterus as it sometimes is called, is not firmly attached nor adherent to any of the bony parts. It is suspended in the pelvic cavity and kept in place by muscles and ligaments. As the muscles and ligaments are elastic, the womb slightly changes its position with different movements of the body. Normally, it is inclined forward, resting on the bladder; so you see, a full bladder will push it backward, while a full rectum and intestines tend to push it forward and downward.

[Illustration: GENERATIVE ORGANS.]

The lower end or mouth of the womb opens into the vagina, a distensible and curved muscular tube, which helps to support the womb and also connects it with the external parts. The vagina is about three and a half inches long. It often is called the birth canal because the baby must pass through it on its way from the womb to the external world.

The two upper openings of the womb lead into the fallopian tubes or oviducts, which are two small muscular tubes leading from the ovaries to the womb. Each one is about four inches long, but the opening through the center in its largest portion is only about as large as a broom straw, while near the womb it narrows down until it will admit only a fine bristle. When the ovum or seed leaves the ovary it must pass through one of these tubes to reach the womb, so you see how necessary it is that they be kept in good condition.

From the end of each tube, but not directly connected with it, is suspended a small almond-shaped body called the ovary. Each ovary is similar in shape and size to an almond, measuring about one and a half inches in length, three-fourths of an inch in width and one-half an inch in thickness. The function or work of the ovaries is to produce, develop and mature the ova (eggs) and to discharge them when fully formed so they may enter the tubes and so find their way to the womb. In every ovary there are several hundred little ovules or eggs in various stages of development. At irregular intervals one of these ovules ripens and leaves the ovary. It passes along the fallopian tube to the womb. Here it remains if it is impregnated or fertilized, and develops into the babe. If not impregnated, it passes off with the menstrual flow. Every twenty-eight days large quantities of blood are sent to the womb, producing a natural congestion. The pressure of this extra blood in the tiny capillaries of the womb stretches and weakens their walls. This allows the blood, which is being sent to the womb to provide nourishment for the ovum if it be impregnated, to pass into the cavity of the womb, then out through the mouth into the vagina, thence to the external parts. This flow is called the menstrual flow. When the flow ceases the mucosa or lining assumes its former state. This process is repeated every month.

Lining the cavity of the abdomen and also folded over the womb, ovaries, tubes and other organs is a thin membrane called the peritoneum. An inflammation of this lining is called peritonitis.

All these organs I have mentioned are situated inside the body out of sight, but there are other organs that are external. You have noticed two longitudinal folds of skin extending from the anus, or external opening of the rectum, to the rounded eminence in front. Their outer surface is covered with hair and their inner surface with glands that secrete a lubricating material. These folds are called the labia majora. Within the labia majora are two smaller folds called the labia minora. These folds meet at their anterior (front) end. At the meeting point you will notice a very small structure which is called the clitoris. This clitoris is very similar in structure to the penis of the male, having a tiny prepuce or foreskin which folds over to protect the sensitive end. Sometimes the foreskin is bound down too tightly, so that instead of being a protection to the parts, it becomes a source of irritation. Then we say the clitoris is hooded and it is necessary to loosen or cut this fold of skin. The operation is similar to that of circumcision in the male.

Just back of the clitoris, within the folds of the labia, is situated the meatus urinarius, or opening leading to the bladder. This aperture does not open directly into the bladder but is connected to it by a tube, about an inch and a half long, called the urethra.

The orifice or external opening of the vagina is situated just back of the meatus urinarius, also within the folds of the labia. In the virgin it is partly closed by a membranous fold called the hymen or maidenhead. The shape and size of the hymen varies greatly in different individuals, sometimes being entirely absent. After marriage it usually persists as notched folds. The presence of an intact hymen is not necessarily a sign of virginity, nor does its absence necessarily indicate defloration. Its congenital absence or absence at the time of birth is known. It sometimes is injured, or may be destroyed by an accident, as by falling astride of an object; again violent exercise may rupture it (horseback riding). Surgical operations or vaginal examinations, roughly conducted, not infrequently cause rupture. Then, too, authentic cases are on record in which prostitutes have had perfectly preserved hymens. It is well known that the use of vaginal astringents may tone up and narrow the vagina and even restore the hymen to a great degree.

The surface between the vaginal orifice and the anus is called the perineum (Do not confuse this with the peritoneum, for they are entirely different). It is this perineum that sometimes becomes torn during childbirth. The vaginal opening does not always stretch sufficiently to allow the passage of the child's head and the great pressure being exerted on the child by the uterine and abdominal muscles pushes it through, causing the tear. (You will understand this better when I explain about the development and birth of the child.) If this tear is repaired immediately no inconvenience usually results but if it is neglected it may produce a series of complications, some of which are falling of the womb, inflammation and even sterility.

Not directly connected with any of the other organs but still associated with them are the breasts. They vary in size at different periods of life, being usually of small size when the girl is young but increasing in size as the generative organs develop. The breasts consist of fatty tissue surrounding milk glands and ducts. During pregnancy they increase in size and become filled with milk. After the menopause (change of life) they ordinarily shrink in size. The ancient Greek statues, such as the Venus de Medici, long regarded as a type of perfect beauty, the Venus of Capua, regarded as the bust of a perfect form, show that the Grecian ideal of the feminine form had small busts. The modern idea seems to have wandered far from the Grecian ideal and many women devote much time and money trying to develop their busts. Perhaps sometime we will give up trying to be so artificial and conform to Nature's ideal.

Nature has constructed the internal female organs so wisely that we seldom need give them much thought. But the external organs do need our attention every day. I told you that the labia secreted a lubricating material which kept the parts moist, but this secretion must not be allowed to accumulate. The scalp secretes an oil that is necessary to the health of the hair but if this and the perspiration are allowed to accumulate the hair has an offensive odor. So it is with the female organs, the parts must be bathed carefully every day. I have been surprised in the past to find how many intelligent women neglect these parts. Women come for an examination, their clothing is scrupulously clean, their bodies show recent care but in the folds of the labia, especially near the clitoris, I find an accumulation of a cheesy-like material which has an odor very offensive to any truly refined woman. Sometimes in public gatherings, I have been seated near a woman with this same offensive odor very noticeable, and I have longed to tell her how to avoid it, for I am sure others must notice the same odor. But even from a physician, in the privacy of the office, women resent any suggestion that they are not thorough in matters of cleanliness. Daily cleansing of these parts is a necessity. At least once a day these parts should be sponged carefully. The labia should be separated and every fold thoroughly cleansed. Occasional vaginal douches also are necessary, for the various secretions often are retained in the folds of the vagina and cause irritation. But in taking a douche one always should remember to have the water warm. Cold water may produce congestion. The virtue of douches (except when taken for medicinal purposes) lies in their cleansing properties and warm water cleanses even better than cold. Many women produce grave disorders by the use of cold douches under the mistaken notion that they are of greater value than hot ones. A douche should be taken at the close of the menstrual period especially.

These female organs should not be the source of worry but they do require as much or even more attention to cleanliness than we give to our mouths or other parts of the body.

CHAPTER II

MENSTRUATION--PUBERTY--MENOPAUSE

The subject of menstruation seems to be troubling several of you. I am sorry that you did not all have the advantage of having this explained at an early age. You might have been saved a great deal of suffering and causeless worry.

By menstruation, or "the monthlies" as it sometimes is called, is meant the monthly hemorrhage that takes place in the uterus or womb during the child-bearing period of the normal woman except during pregnancy and lactation, when it nearly always is suspended. The child-bearing period commences at the age of puberty and ends with the menopause (change of life).

Puberty is the period of maturing of the sexual organs. It occurs about the age of twelve, although there may be considerable variation as to this. It extends over a period of several years. As a rule, girls mature earlier in warm climates than in cold and in cities than in country districts. The signs of the approach of this period are the growth of hair on the pubes and other parts of the body, the enlargement of the breasts, a general rounding and increased grace of the body, the development of the pelvis so that the hips become more prominent, and a change in the mental qualities of the child, the girl naturally becoming more retiring. The menstrual function usually is not established at once, there being premonitory symptoms of a vague nature. There may be, at first, only a slight discharge of mucus tinged with blood, later the normal menstrual flow will be established.

During this period of puberty there are great changes taking place in the girl's internal organs. This change and development requires considerable of the girl's strength and naturally influences her nervous system. It is for this reason that a girl at this period of her life should not be subjected to any great exertion, either physical or mental. She should have plenty of light, healthful exercise in the open air, but should not indulge in any very violent exercise. A little care at this time often will save her years of suffering. As the nervous system is greatly affected at this period there should be no great mental strain. In fact, if the girl shows many nervous symptoms, it may be wise to take her out of school for a year so that her strength may be used as Nature requires it. As a rule, too much work is required in school at this age. The school duties should be lessened and the girl allowed to rest a day or two during her menstrual period. The girl at this age should not attempt to accomplish as much work or study as the boy does. Her time at this period might better be occupied in learning the rudiments of housekeeping and home-making. Then, when her body has become developed, her strength can be spared and can be well used in the development of her mind. If the nervous strain too common at this age could be relieved we would have fewer nervous women and a healthier and happier posterity.

As puberty approaches, a mother should give her daughter adequate information so that she should not be frightened at the first appearance of the menstrual flow, nor take any risks at this period. Menstruation is the sign of the possibility of motherhood. If properly taught this fact, every girl will be glad she menstruates and will want to be careful during the period. On account of lack of early instruction, many a girl obtains wrong ideas regarding this function and it produces in her a feeling of repugnance. She should be taught the reasons for observing prudence during the menstrual period. The possible lifelong invalidism that may result should be pointed out. A woman owes it to herself to take good care of herself during her menstrual periods. For two or three days at least she should avoid any unnecessary strain, lie down and rest as much as possible and not worry over school or other duties.

Especial attention should be paid to cleanliness during this period. A sponge bath taken in a warm room is not injurious and unpleasant odors can be avoided by sponging the parts with a warm antiseptic solution upon changing the cloth. Every woman should be provided with a circular girdle cut upon the bias so it may be elastic, and provided with tabs to which to pin the folded cloth. She also should have a supply of sanitary cloths made of absorbent cotton-fabric, or pads made of absorbent cotton enclosed in gauze. The latter especially are convenient for the girl who is obliged to room away from home, for they may be burned and the cost of new ones is no greater than the laundry of cloths. These pads or cloths should be changed at least twice a day. It also is necessary that one should bathe the parts in warm water with each change, as unpleasant odors can thereby be avoided. At the close of each period she should take a bath and change all clothing. One cannot be too careful about these matters so essential to cleanliness. It is surprising how many women neglect these important matters. The erroneous idea that bathing of any sort at this time may have disastrous results accounts for much of this neglect. If proper care is taken warm sponge baths cannot be injurious.

A woman in normal health should not suffer at the menstrual period. She normally will have a feeling of lassitude and disinclination for any great mental or physical work, perhaps accompanied by a slight feeling of uneasiness in the pelvic region. Because so many women do suffer at these periods it often is considered as "natural" and allowed to continue.

The phenomena often noted at the menstrual period are,--pains in various parts of the body, hot flashes, chilliness and various hysterical symptoms. A few days before menstruation commences there may be various nervous symptoms, as irritability and a disinclination for any exertion. Dark circles often appear under the eyes and the breasts become enlarged and painful. A sense of fullness and oppression may be felt in the head.

Any severe pain or profuse flow during the period or a discharge between periods indicates a weakened or diseased condition and should not be neglected, for it sooner or later will affect the whole system. A woman suffering from female diseases not only is unable to perform her work in a normal manner but the pale skin, dark circles under the eyes and drawn haggard look which accompany these conditions rob her of her charm of physical excellence.

The menstrual flow appears, as a rule, every twenty-eight days, although the length of time varies with the individual. The average duration is five days, but varies from three to seven. The flow consists of blood from the uterine mucosa (lining of the womb) together with small quantities of mucus. The color generally is dark at first while later it becomes more pale. Women in poor health often have a pale discharge. There always is a faint odor to the menstrual flow, which has been likened to the odor of marigolds. The quantity varies with the individual. Usually fleshy girls flow more than thin ones and dark complexioned ones than light ones. The average quantity is four to six fluid ounces. The time between the periods is required by the uterus or womb to first restore the lining and then prepare it for the reception of the ovum. Every month one or more ova (eggs) leave the ovary, pass to the uterus and, if not impregnated, pass off with the menstrual flow. The material prepared for the reception of the ovum is used to nourish the new life if pregnancy occurs, but when it does not, this surplus passes off in the form of the menstrual flow.

The menopause or change of life is the end of the child-bearing period of a woman's life. The average age at which it occurs is forty-six, although there is a great difference as to this. In some women it has been known to occur as early as the thirtieth year, while in others it does not come until the fifty-fifth year. As a rule, a woman who commences to menstruate at an early age continues to do so until a late age, while with a woman who commences to menstruate late, the change comes early. At this period of a woman's life, there are numerous changes taking place in the body. The ovaries and uterus atrophy or shrink in size, and cease to functionate. The nervous system is being readjusted to meet the changed conditions. One symptom of the approach of this period is irregularity in menstruation; sometimes several periods are missed, then the menstrual flow appears normally for several months and then disappears again. Often the woman complains of hot flashes, cramps in the limbs and other parts of the body. These are caused by the attempts to readjust the nervous system to the altered conditions. A great many women worry unnecessarily, for there is no especial danger at this time unless the body has been neglected previously and a diseased condition is present. But the body needs a little extra care, just as it did at puberty. So many women break down their health by worrying at this period over what might happen. The best plan for every woman, as soon as she perceives the approach of this period, is to go to a reliable physician and have a thorough examination. Then if there are any neglected tears or chronic inflammations they can be corrected and danger removed. If a person were to cross a deep lake and had any doubts regarding the worthiness of the vessel provided for his use, he would be very foolish if he did not have a trained boat-builder examine his vessel and repair any weak places. It is just as important for a woman about to cross this period of her life to go to a trained repairer of bodies and have him correct any weak places.

The various changes taking place consume so much of the woman's strength that she requires an extra amount of rest and cannot use up as much energy in working as at other periods of her life. The ordinary woman does not realize the need of extra rest during this period and so continues her usual work. Then the extra drain on her nervous system shows itself in various forms. The disturbances sometimes are productive of so much discomfort and so often are exaggerated beyond physiological limits that the patient is impelled to seek relief and often requires a physician's attention. Puberty or the period of development extends over several years, so the menopause or period of atrophy extends over a period of from three to five years. If a woman relaxes and allows the changes to proceed naturally she need have no cause to worry, but she must remember that rest from continual strain is necessary during this period. Freedom from care, relaxation of physical and mental effort, regular periods of complete rest once or twice a day, a reduction of the diet and regulation of the bowels should be the first principles of treatment. Then--do not worry but occupy the mind with happy thoughts.

CHAPTER III

DISEASES OF THE FEMALE ORGANS

So much of the suffering among women is unnecessary, being due to the neglect of the little things, so much ill health can be relieved by attention to a few simple hygienic measures, that I think it wise to describe some of the most common disorders of the female organs, and to explain their symptoms so that you would not ignorantly neglect them, if you should be so unfortunate as to contract any.

The most common diseases of the female organs may be classed as displacements, inflammations and tumors.

On account of its lack of strong attachment, the womb is very easily displaced. When from any cause the womb is congested and heavy the extra weight stretches the supporting muscles and ligaments, which then allow it to fall out of place. It also may be displaced by a sudden fall, by jumping or other strenuous exercise. As the womb normally is heavier at the menstrual period than at any other time and as there is a natural congestion then, it is more easily displaced at that time than during any other part of the month. This is one reason why one should be careful not to take strenuous exercise at the menstrual period.

The most common displacement, or the most common way for the womb to tip, is backwards and at the same time it usually falls downward. You remember, the rectum is directly back of the womb, so, if the womb is tipped backwards, it presses against the rectum. This tends to prevent the feces, or bowel movement, from passing out naturally and helps to produce constipation. The womb, pressing against the rectum, also presses on the blood vessels which are very numerous there. This pressure on the blood vessels prevents the blood from leaving them. If it is held there, it causes the blood vessels to dilate in order to be large enough to contain it. We call this enlarged portion of the vein a blood tumor. These tumors or dilated blood vessels of the rectum are called hemorrhoids or piles. I will explain these more thoroughly when I talk to you about constipation.

The womb may tip forward, pressing on the bladder and causing a frequent desire to urinate. More rarely it is tipped to one side. It then tends to pull on the ovaries and produce pain and various nervous symptoms.

The womb may fall downward, pressing against both the bladder and rectum and dragging the ovaries and tubes out of their natural positions. Sometimes it even protrudes from the vagina. Any falling or displacement of the womb pulls on the tubes and ovaries, often producing an inflammation. This inflammation should not be allowed to continue, as it may become serious, even extending to the peritoneum and producing peritonitis. The nerves of the uterus are very closely connected with the spinal nerves, therefore, any displacement reacts through them and may produce headache and backache, which are the common accompaniments of any uterine disorder.

[Illustration: KNEE-CHEST POSITION]

One of the most simple and yet efficacious treatments to correct a displacement downward and backward is to assume the knee-chest position for a few moments morning and evening after the clothing has been removed. In the knee-chest position, the patient kneels on the bed, then bends forward until her chest touches the bed; the back slopes down and the thighs should be at right angles with the bed. This position allows the various organs to fall forward and toward the upper part of the body, the pressure on the uterus is relieved and it assumes its natural position. This treatment, persisted in, will relieve nearly every case which has not some other disorder connected with it. If every woman would assume this position for a few minutes once or twice a week, just before retiring, she would be greatly benefited; for the majority of women have a slight falling of the womb, which then presses on the rectal and other nerves causing various nervous symptoms.

The womb and ovaries are surrounded by a dense network of nerves and blood vessels, making them very liable to congestion. Tight clothing or improperly fitted clothing causes pressure and interferes with the circulation. I believe that a large percentage of the objections to the corset originated from women wearing improperly fitted corsets which pushed the organs out of place. A corset fitted to the wearer is not injurious and serves as a support. Overwork, catching cold and excesses may produce a congestion which is one stage of inflammation. The most common symptoms of inflammation of the womb are pain in the pelvic region, a dull backache, especially across the hips, and a vaginal discharge called leucorrhoea (whites). Any leucorrhoea shows a disordered condition which should be corrected. It may be simply of a catarrhal nature, due to pressure or cold, or it may indicate a more serious condition, as the presence of one of the black plagues. Whenever a woman notices a vaginal discharge, it is a wise plan to go at once to a reliable physician, find out what is the cause and nature and then take measures to correct it. In the beginning a very little treatment, such as hot douches, may be all that is required, while if untreated the condition may become serious, as you will understand when I explain about the black plagues.

Any disorder of the uterus or ovaries reacts through the nerves upon other parts of the body and may produce various symptoms such as general weakness, headaches and backaches. This drain on the system often is shown by dark circles under the eyes, pale skin and a drawn, haggard expression. All these tend to rob a woman of her charm of physical excellence, and none of us wish to lose that; for it is natural for all women to wish to appear attractive.

One of the most common of the so-called female disorders, which seems to be the lot of the majority of women, is dysmenorrhoea or painful menstruation. This is not a disease in itself, but the symptom of various disorders. A woman in normal health should not suffer at her menstrual period; so if she does suffer it shows there is something wrong. The natural thing for anyone to do who had dysmenorrhoea would be first to find the cause of this pain and then take measures to correct it. It may be due to displacements, inflammations or tumors; it may be due to a contraction of the mouth of the womb which does not dilate sufficiently to allow the menstrual discharge to flow freely. It may be due to neuralgia or rheumatism of the uterus or ovaries. Pain always indicates an unnatural condition. It is the cry of tortured nerves. The cause should be determined by a competent physician and then measures taken immediately to restore the normal condition.

One who suffers from dysmenorrhoea should try to plan her work so that she may rest the first day of her menstrual period, and, if possible, the preceding day. Absolute rest in bed at this time is beneficial. A hot sitz bath, hot foot bath or hot vaginal douche taken just previous to the commencement of the period will aid in relieving the congestion and thus lessen the pain. After the flow has started hot foot baths and hot applications to the abdomen may be used. Hot drinks also may be taken, but one should not get in the habit of using any drug at this time. Hot ginger tea will do as much good as one prepared with some habit-forming drug. Many of the remedies advertised as a cure for this condition are composed chiefly of alcohol, and, although they may give a temporary relief, the benefit is not permanent. Careful attention to diet and exercise, with regular hours of sleep, are essential points to be considered if one would be free from this disagreeable trouble.

Another symptom which often causes much alarm to the patient is amenorrhoea or deficient or scanty menstruation. This may result from fear, worry, catching cold or to an enlargement of the womb. It also is one of the first symptoms of pregnancy. Sometimes it indicates an impoverished condition of the blood and shows the need of a general building up of the system. This is true especially in young girls who have what is called chlorosis or green sickness. These girls are pale, weak, sometimes having a greenish cast to their complexions. They need good care and nourishing food and plenty of light, outdoor exercise.

In young girls I sometimes find an irritation of the vagina which causes pain. This may be due to the retention of secretions in the vagina. The general idea that only married women have leucorrhoea, or whites, is fallacious. Virgins may have it. The usual cause is catching cold at the menstrual period. Another delusion is that these girls should not take douches for fear they might injure the hymen. This is erroneous, for douches are necessary in the treatment of this condition and, except in very rare cases, a douche can be taken with an especially small douche point without injury to the parts. There normally must be a small opening in the hymen to permit the passage of the menstrual flow. If a small douche point is used no harm will result.

When I talked to you about the structure of the external generative organs, I mentioned the clitoris and explained that sometimes the prepuce or foreskin is bound down, or is too tight, so that the natural secretions are retained under it and produce an irritation; that the operation for the unhooding of the clitoris is very similiar to that of circumcision in the male and is performed for similar causes. Many a woman who has been nervous all her life, owes her condition to a hooded clitoris, which a very simple operation would correct. A hooded clitoris also may have something to do with the immoral life of some girls. The other day I received a letter from an aged physician who, in discussing the tendency to immoral practices, says: "You say in one of your articles, 'What is the remedy? Educate!' Well, perhaps, but if you would let me circumcise the girl early in life, I believe it would be more certain." There is considerable truth in his statement. A hooded clitoris produces a constant irritation which tends to lead to habits of self-abuse and perhaps immorality.

The other common disorder which I named at first is a tumor. Tumors are any unnatural growth. They may form in any part of the body, but just now we will speak only of those affecting the internal female organs. Tumors may form in the cavity of the womb, in its walls or on the outside of it. The common symptoms are an enlargement of the abdomen accompanied usually by pain due to pressure on the nerves. There also may be some hemorrhage at other than the regular menstrual periods.

Sometimes the ovaries are diseased and become enlarged, tender and filled with fluid. Then they are spoken of as cystic tumors or as cysts. The tubes may become inflamed and filled with pus. The most common cause of these pus tubes is one of the black plagues. With all these tumors the treatment usually is to remove the tumor and sometimes the entire organ. In a few cases it is possible that the fluid or other contents of the tumor may be absorbed, if the general health and circulation are improved. In some cases we find what is called a phantom tumor. There really is no tumor, although the symptoms may be such that even reliable physicians are misled. The symptoms are due to a nervous condition. These phantom tumors have given many a quack a reputation for removing tumors without the use of the knife.

A carcinoma or cancer is a malignant tumor, that is, one that tends to grow worse and to reappear if it apparently is removed. The reappearance may be in the same place or in an entirely different portion of the body. Cancer of the uterus is not uncommon in women. It frequently follows neglect of some injury. For example, it will appear on the site of an unrepaired tear. It most commonly comes after the menopause. The change that is undergone at that time seems to stir things up and bring to light any neglected injury. This is another reason why every woman at the menopause should undergo a thorough examination and have any defect repaired, thus avoiding much of the possibility of trouble. A frequent symptom of carcinoma of the uterus is hemorrhage at irregular times after the menopause. Any woman who has such a condition would be wise if she immediately repaired to a physician and determined the cause of the hemorrhage. In the beginning it is possible to remove a cancer, but later it becomes so involved in the surrounding structures that its removal is impossible.

You may think I am trying to increase business for the physicians but in reality my advice, if taken, would lessen their practice. It is another application of "a stitch in time saves nine." In the beginning almost all these diseases can be corrected with very little trouble, while if neglected the process is much slower. The probabilities are that the doctor will have the case later, if not consulted early, but instead of a few office treatments he will have an expensive operation. So, you see, I really am trying to save you doctors' bills when I urge early and thorough examinations. There is a peculiar thing about the human race. A machine will get out of order and the owner will send for an expert machinist to repair it--not attempting to patch it up himself. But when these bodies of ours, the most wonderful and complicated of machines, get out of repair we try to patch them up ourselves or try various remedies recommended by those who know worse than nothing about the physical machinery. Then we think we are saving doctors' bills, when at the same time we are spending twice as much on questionable repairs--patent medicines, which often do more harm than good. Frequently they contain stimulants which produce a mythical improvement but leave the system worse off than before.

CHAPTER IV

CONSTIPATION--HEMORRHOIDS

A regular daily movement of the bowels is necessary to health. Much of the illness in the world might have been avoided if the victims had taken better care of the excretory organs. One of the first questions a physician asks a patient is, "How are your bowels, do they move regularly every day?" In some cases that is the first time the patient has thought of them, and he has to think some time before he can remember just when and how often his bowels did move. Then perhaps he is not sure. In a great many cases it is a routine practice with physicians to give a "good cleaning out," that is, to give a thorough laxative. Many times this is all the treatment required and in other cases it only is combined with a little intestinal antiseptic to further carry out the cleaning process.

The most common cause of constipation is irregularity in going to the toilet. When the desire for defecation comes, we are too busy and postpone it until some more convenient time, which time may be too late. Nature is the best judge as to when the bowels are ready to be emptied. If we do not obey her call, we must take the consequences. When the waste material is ready to be voided, it is in a semi-fluid state, but, if it remains in the intestines too long the water is absorbed and the waste material is left in a hard mass which is expelled with difficulty. Not only that, but the desire to expel it soon passes. Nature, finding we do not respond to her call, ceases to notify us.

If the waste material is allowed to remain in the bowels, not only the water is absorbed but with it some of the poisons from the waste material, which are taken up by the blood and carried to all parts of the system, causing a great deal of trouble and pain. This absorption of toxins (poisons) causes headache, loss of appetite, a sense of depression and a lack of energy.

The pressure of the hard material on the tender tissues of the rectum causes hemorrhoids or piles, by irritating the tissues and causing a congestion. Hemorrhoids are enlarged veins which have been so irritated and filled with extra blood that they have lost their power to contract. These enlarged veins may remain inside the rectum and then are known as internal piles. Sometimes they protrude externally and then are known as external piles. Frequently they become tender and cause a great deal of pain. In some cases one of the little veins becomes so engorged with blood that it bursts and allows the contained blood to escape. This is known as bleeding piles. For mild cases of hemorrhoids (piles) the treatment is to correct the accompanying constipation, then take an enema or injection of warm water morning and evening, using the water as hot as can be borne and allowing it to run in and out the rectum for some time. Following this, an astringent and soothing lotion should be applied.

Constipation may be caused by retroversion of the uterus. If the uterus is tipped backwards it presses on the rectum, preventing the passage of the feces (bowel movement). This pressure also causes hemorrhoids. In this case the treatment is to correct the displacement. In many cases all that is necessary is to take the knee-chest position for a few minutes night and morning.

Always in the treatment of constipation, the first item is to discover the cause. We have noted that the chief cause is irregularity in going to the toilet, therefore, the first measure to be taken in the treatment is regularity in going to the toilet. Choose a convenient hour, usually right after breakfast, and always go to the toilet at that time no matter if there is a desire or not. At first there may be no natural movement but if you persist, your efforts will be rewarded. For the first few days it is well to take an enema of warm, soapy water at this time. Every day take exercise that will strengthen the muscles of the abdomen. Bending forward and touching the toes with the fingers without bending the knees is one valuable exercise. This should be done ten or twelve times morning and evening. A daily brisk walk in the fresh air is another good exercise. Fruit or figs eaten with the meals or a glass of water taken before breakfast and upon retiring often proves very beneficial in relieving a tendency to constipation. There is an old saying, "An apple or two before going to bed, and the doctor will go begging for his bread." This really is a practical idea and more nearly true than many old sayings.

Cathartics or laxatives should not be taken except for an occasional dose or during illness upon the advice of a physician. So common is the practice of taking daily laxatives that it has become a "national curse"! People do not realize that they are slaves to this habit, so they continue to take their daily doses of "teas" or "waters." In many cases a patient will tell his physician that his bowels are "all right," that they move every day. Further questionings reveal the fact that he is in the habit of taking some laxative frequently. The bowels are not "all right" if any laxative is required.

Massage of the abdomen usually is very beneficial in treating constipation. It acts by stimulating the muscles and should be given at set times in the day but never until two hours after any meal. The various vibrators act in the same manner as massage. In any massage of the abdomen the thighs should be flexed, as this relaxes the abdominal muscles.

Enemas or injections of warm water may be taken occasionally and then are beneficial, but if long continued are injurious by reason of their irritating effect. At times, when the stomach and intestines have been over-loaded with irritating material, an enema is one of the quickest measures for relief. In obstinate constipation two or three ounces of warm olive oil injected slowly into the rectum at night and allowed to remain until morning will soften the waste material so it can be evacuated easily in the morning.

Constipation never should be neglected as it carries in its train a long line of disorders, as hemorrhoids (piles), abscesses, and intestinal obstruction.

Indigestion and constipation frequently are bosom friends. How often indigestion is a result of nervous strain is perhaps seldom realized. A business man eats his lunch and other meals in a hurry, with his mind on his business. His energies are being consumed by his brain and very little is left to be used in the digestion of his food. One never should eat when tired and nervous. Take a few moments' absolute rest before meals. If possible lie down and relax all muscles for a few moments. Then eat your meal slowly and if possible have some pleasant companion who will talk with you on subjects not connected with your business cares. You will be surprised to note the improvement in your digestion and incidentally in your tendency to constipation.

For the noon meal, office workers should eat only light and easily digested food. Eat your heaviest meal after the work for the day is finished and the blood which has been required by the brain can be spared to the stomach. People doing manual labor that requires physical strength need, and can digest, a heavy noonday meal but the requirements of the brain workers are quite different.

Many girls break down on account of lack of sufficient nourishment. Coffee and rolls for breakfast, ice cream and rolls for lunch and a sandwich and coffee for dinner is not sufficient food for any working girl. And yet that is about the diet of hundreds of girls. Often it is impossible for her to provide more, for when a girl must pay for her board, room, clothes and laundry from her salary of five or six dollars a week, sufficient food becomes an impossibility. Many girls actually are slowly starving on this account. When the wheels of progress make it possible for every working girl to have a comfortable home and sufficient nourishing food many of the social problems will right themselves.

CHAPTER V

THE BLACK PLAGUES

I promised to explain to you what I meant by the black plagues. It is strange when anything is as widely spread as are these diseases that so few people know anything about them, or realize their importance. At one time epidemics of typhoid fever were regarded as a revelation of the wrath of God. Now we know they are due to carelessness and lack of sanitation. It is the same with the sufferings of women. We used to think it was a dispensation of Providence if a woman were compelled to undergo an operation. Now we know it usually is due to someone's lack of care, to a desecration of Nature's teachings.

I remember when I was quite young hearing mention made of a "bad disease." Concerning the nature of this disease I was ignorant but I gathered the idea that it was some terrible disease which was contracted only by the most depraved of mortals. How little I suspected its widely-spread distribution, and how little I dreamed that among my acquaintances might be any afflicted with these diseases! nor did I dream of the danger of innocent contagion. Since then I have learned what these diseases were. Now we call them the black plagues, because, owing to the prejudice of the majority, we dare not use their correct names generally. I have no doubt you will be as surprised and shocked as I was at the things I am going to impart to you.

By black plagues we mean the two diseases spoken of by physicians as the venereal diseases, because they usually are contracted during sexual intercourse.

The most common of these diseases is gonorrhoea, or clap, as it often is called by men. How common it is may be judged by a statement made by a professor to his class in the medical college that at least eighty per cent. of the men in the world have contracted it sometime during their lives. Even the most conservative give the estimate as sixty per cent.

The prevalent idea common among men that it is no worse than a cold--a mere annoyance that all men must expect and endure sometime--is lamentable. The persistence of the disease in the deeper structures long after it outwardly is cured leads to unexpected communication of it to women, among whom may be the young wife. As a result she enters upon a period of ill-health that ultimately may compel the mutilation of her body by a surgical operation to save her life. Much of the surgery performed upon the female organs has been rendered necessary by disease contracted from the husband.

A few little germs of this disease left on even the external organs may find their way up through the vagina to the uterus or womb. Here they may produce an inflammation of the lining of the womb, causing severe pain and other symptoms, such as profuse discharge. The germs may go farther, or the inflammation may extend from the uterus to the tubes. When we consider that the passage through the tubes is only about as large as a broom straw, we see what serious trouble may result. The tubes become enlarged and filled with pus. The opening from the tubes to the uterus becomes closed, so there is no way for the pus to escape. The accumulation of pus or the products of septic inflammation stretch the walls of the tubes until the little nerves in the walls cry out in rebellion. The pain becomes so great and the reflex symptoms are so aggravated that finally the woman resorts to the only relief,--an operation for the removal of the tubes.

When we consider that the ovule, the human egg, must travel through these tubes to reach the uterus and, if they are destroyed, has no other way of reaching the womb and, if it cannot reach the womb and be impregnated, cannot develop into the babe, then we realize how this disease is dooming women to childless lives,--women whose natural instincts and desires cry out for motherhood. When we consider the factors that promote race suicide we must not forget this important one. Even though the woman refuses an operation, or in a case in which the inflammation is not so severe and is reduced until she is nearly free from pain, the result may be the same, for the tubes may remain closed permanently.

The closure of the tubes is not the only result that may follow the course of this disease. The infection may extend into the peritoneal cavity causing peritonitis, which so often results in the untimely death of the woman. Here let me say that not all cases of peritonitis or of inflammation of the womb, tubes or ovaries are due to this infection. There are other infections, other germs, that may produce similar results. These germs may reach the organs in various ways. Sometimes the woman herself is to blame and sometimes we can blame no one. Inflammation of these organs may result from pressure of clothing, colds, excitement, overwork, pregnancies, excesses or neglect. The inflammation may spread to these organs from an inflamed appendix or other neighboring organs.

Supposing, though, following this disease the tubes are not entirely closed and the woman becomes pregnant. There is still the danger that during labor the baby's eyes will become infected and may become permanently blind. It is estimated that seventy per cent. of the blindness in the world has this cause. How does this produce blindness? Some few germs of this disease have remained in the vagina or birth canal and as the baby passes along the canal they enter its eyes. They are so very strong and work so rapidly that they can cause total blindness within three days. This fact is so well known by physicians that at the present time all reliable physicians pay especial attention to the newborn baby's eyes, cleansing them with an antiseptic solution immediately after birth. This precaution doubtless has saved the eyes of thousands of babies. This is one of the reasons why it is dangerous to employ an uneducated person at the time of labor. Even though she may have assisted at hundreds of births yet often she is ignorant of the many dangers and of the precautions that should be taken in every case.

Even adults may become blind from this infection. The disease is carried to the eyes by polluted fingers or towels. In a few hours the eyes become inflamed, pus forms, and unless heroic measures are taken, the eyesight is soon destroyed.

In female children the vagina may become infected through the use of tainted sponges, wash cloths, etc. An innocent girl may thus carelessly acquire the disease. For this reason, we see how necessary it is to caution girls never to use public towels or wash cloths that have been used by another person. Even in the home, every member of the family should have his exclusive towel and wash cloth.

The symptoms of gonorrhoea that often are noted first are a profuse discharge from the vagina, usually creamy or yellowish in color. This discharge is of such a nature that frequently it excoriates the external parts so that they become very tender and inflamed. Backache, especially across the hips, is a common accompaniment of this disease. There may be general soreness in the pelvic region. If a woman suspects she has contracted this disease, she should go immediately to some reliable physician; for at first the disease may affect only the vagina but, if neglected, may extend to the uterus and tubes. In its early stages it may be cured by prompt treatment, but the majority of women postpone treatment until it is too late.

The other loathsome disease, syphilis, infects the blood and therefore all parts of the body. While under proper treatment it is not dangerous to life in the earlier years, yet the possibilities of conveying the contagion are numerous. In the second stage, which lasts for a number of weeks, the mucous patches in the mouth are a source of danger. In this stage the disease may be conveyed by a kiss or through the medium of the public drinking cup, towel, or anything that comes in contact with the virus. It may be contracted by a babe from a wet-nurse or the nurse may contract it from the babe.

The most serious results of this disease appear years after its initial appearance, when the individual has been lulled into a false sense of security by long freedom from its outward symptoms. Many of the obscure cases of stomach or nerve trouble may be traced to this disease. The results not only affect the man, but, should he marry and have children, his innocent babes may come into the world with an inherited taint. These children seldom live to reach adult life and their lives usually are burdensome and full of misery. They may be deformed or be continually afflicted with ulcers or other horrible manifestations of the disease. I will explain this more thoroughly when I speak of heredity.

Many of the disastrous effects of these diseases might have been prevented if they had been properly treated in their early stages. Ignorance as to the nature and probable disastrous effects, if neglected, prevents many a person from procuring proper treatment. It is a common practice among men afflicted with these diseases to try various remedies recommended by their friends or by the druggist. It is strange that a person who would not think of trying to treat himself for smallpox or other contagious disease will do so with these diseases. With women, the cause of their neglect is a failure to realize the importance of the symptoms. Unfortunately women have grown to think that various female ills are their lot in life which must be endured and regarded as a dispensation of Providence instead of being considered an error in living that must be corrected the same as any other disease. Some commence treatment but neglect it as soon as the noticeable symptoms have disappeared. It generally is considered among physicians that the treatment of syphilis should be continued for at least three years after contracting the disease in order to remove all traces from the blood.

It is a deplorable fact that the prevalence of these diseases might have been prevented by proper instruction of young boys. No man ever willfully contracted one of these diseases. Statistics tell us that the majority of victims contract them before their twentieth year, before the boy has learned anything of their dangers or perhaps of their existence. If these patients received the right treatment immediately and continued it until the disease had been eradicated the results would have been less serious. Here, too, lack of early and proper instruction is shown; for these immature boys do not realize the necessity for prompt and wise treatment, or are misled by unscrupulous persons. I shall talk to you again on this subject, for many of you will have sons and you must know the dangers that beset them, so they can be prepared.

CHAPTER VI

FAKE MEDICAL ADVICE FOR WOMEN

One young lady wrote me, "Recently I read that imperfectly developed ovaries might be a reason why some women do not have children. I have the symptoms which the article said indicated imperfect development. Does this necessarily mean that I never can have a baby? I seem to be healthy. I am twenty-one years old. I was to have been married in three months but now I do not know what to do. 'My boy' loves children as I do. It seems as though I cannot give him up, yet it surely is not honorable to marry him if I find that I never will have a little one, without telling him. Please tell me what to do."

The probabilities are that this girl's ovaries are perfectly normal and that the article mentioned was an advertisement of some medical house which, by misleading statements, endeavors to induce women to take their treatment. There are many women who suffer a great deal mentally, and this in turn reflects on their physical health because of just such articles.

It has been said that we are a nation of dupes and the advertisements carried in some of the papers would indicate the truth of this statement. No manufacturer is going to advertise anything that does not sell well and bring a considerable profit. Men are not so altruistic as to be in business just for the good of humanity. The majority are in business for the money to be obtained from it. Somehow, women are very susceptible to the arts of these greedy manufacturers. A company commences to make a patent medicine and then, in order to derive any profits from the investment, large quantities of the preparation must be sold. In order to accomplish this they must convince possible buyers of their need of this particular treatment. The company employs an agent to write an advertisement, perhaps in the shape of an article purporting to be written by someone much interested in the human race. This advertisement or article describes some disease which may be cured by this one remedy. As there might not be enough people who know they have this given disease to make a profit for the manufacturer, it becomes his business to convince others that they have this disease. Therefore, he proceeds to enumerate a great many symptoms which he says indicate this disease. Perhaps they might! But they are just as likely to indicate any one of half a dozen other things. He details enough symptoms so that some are recognized by nearly every woman as relating to her condition, so she jumps to the conclusion that she has that certain disease and buys a bottle of the medicine.

If you will study the large medical advertisements that appeal especially to women you will notice that they all have certain symptoms enumerated. No matter if the remedy advertised is for the kidneys, the bowels, or exclusively for women, the same symptoms are claimed to indicate the need of that certain remedy. One of the symptoms most commonly given is backache. Of course! For nearly every person has a backache at some time. It may be due to a strain, to rheumatism of the lumbar muscles (lumbago), to constipation, to a displacement, or to numerous other conditions. No one can tell the cause who is not properly prepared to do so and who is not fully acquainted with the physical condition. The sewing machine runs hard and perhaps makes a noise. It requires a mechanic who is familiar with the mechanism of the machine to find the cause of the trouble. So it is with the human body. It requires a mechanic who is familiar with the structure of the body to discover the cause of the trouble. And yet people will continue to pour into their bodies drugs, harmless and otherwise, that are manufactured by some enterprising firm and then advertised by an expert who knows nothing of disease except a few symptoms common to almost all diseases.

The patent medicine consumers seldom realize the nature of the medicine they take. Because some man, desirous of selling his remedy, claims it will be beneficial, they rush in and buy. To one who knows the true nature of some of these remedies, many laughable instances are visible. One man recently discovered that a temperance agitator was daily dosing herself with a certain tonic which was known to contain a larger percentage of alcohol than did the beverages she was denouncing so ardently.

Patent medicines may benefit some, but in the majority of cases, the consumer is like a man who boards the nearest street-car hoping it will take him to his destination. It may! But it is just as likely to take him in the opposite direction.

Some people become veritable drug fiends, slaves to certain drugs without in the least realizing their condition. How many are slaves to certain laxatives or headache powders! With them the daily dose of "harmless" teas or waters or even of pills cannot be neglected. And yet such a person would be indignant at the suggestion that she was the victim of a drug habit. What are drugs, anyhow? The majority are simply extracts of herbs and vegetables. And yet people imagine that they are avoiding the use of drugs and medicines when they take "simple herb remedies, prepared at home."

Another lure of the advertiser is to state that all letters are "strictly confidential and answered by women only." Perhaps they are! But he neglects to add that the women who answer these letters are simply stenographers with no medical knowledge, employed to write according to dictation, that the letters are all written according to certain forms which have been dictated by the manager. A short time ago a young woman wrote me regarding her condition. Among other things, she said she had written to a certain woman whose name is much advertised by a patent medicine concern and that this woman had written her advice that had caused her to worry over her condition. Poor, deluded girl! How was she to know that the woman in question had been dead many years and that the business was carried on by her son and other men.

If you are ill do not be misled by these unscrupulous advertisers. Do not waste your time and money on remedies that may be entirely unsuited to your condition.

CHAPTER VII

THE MARRIAGE RELATION

As several of you expect to be married soon I think it would be well to talk briefly about the cause of so much unhappiness in marriage.

It has been estimated that only about five per cent. of all marriages are successful. Is this true, and if true, why? If five per cent. made a success of marriage, why could not the other ninety-five? Marriage is a science to be studied by the prospective bride and groom in order that they may be ranked with the five per cent. and not make a failure of their married life. Few would enter the marriage relation if convinced that it would be a failure. The prospective bride looks around among her acquaintances and sees the lack of true happiness, thinks that her case will be an exception, that her marriage will turn out all right and then goes blindly ahead into the new life without any preparation.

A large percentage of the unhappiness among married couples comes through a misunderstanding of the marital relations. A great deal of this is due to ignorance on the part of the bride and thoughtlessness on the part of the husband. This is partly due to defective education during childhood in regard to the sexes. The training of boys and girls in this matter is very different. Knowledge pertaining to the sexual life is talked over very freely among boys, so that by the time the boy is of a marriageable age he is pretty well posted. With girls it is quite different. It would be considered very immodest for a girl to discuss such matters. She does not feel free even to talk with her mother or other adviser, and so she goes to the altar ignorant of many things she should know. Then during the first few days of married life this knowledge so overwhelms her and often gives her such a severe shock that it leaves a lasting impression. She has no way of knowing that her husband is just like other men. She is liable to regard him as a brute and resent his attentions.

Such a condition of affairs is altogether wrong, but the girl is not to be blamed. Had she been taught what to expect, much of the unhappiness of married life might have been avoided. If taught correctly, the girl should regard the sexual act as the culmination of true love. It should be regarded as something sacred, something that makes her and her husband as one. Fortunate indeed is the girl whose husband realizes this lack of knowledge and gently leads her to desire the fulfillment of love. Unfortunate is the girl whose husband regards this act only as the gratification of animal passions-- something it is a wife's duty to endure as such.

Passion or sex sense is a sign of maturity. It is the calling for a mate. All animals have this sense and nearly all animals have a mating season. The billing and cooing of the birds in the springtime is an expression of this sense--the love sense. It is possessed by every little insect. Only by knowing their habits do we see the expression of it. This sense is nothing of which one should be ashamed. It was God-given for a divine purpose.

In the study of plants we learn that the pollen or male element must unite with the ovum or female element in order to produce the seed that will develop into the new plant. The same fact is true of the human race. Before pregnancy can take place there must be a meeting and fusion of the vital elements of the two sexes. This fertilization of the ovum or joining of the male and female elements is called conception. It is brought about by coitus, by means of which the semen of the male is deposited in the vagina of the female. This act is called insemination, although conception does not follow unless the ovum and spermatozoon (life-giving element of the semen) come together and unite. When this occurs the woman conceives and enters upon a period of pregnancy. The time at which conception is least likely to occur is from the seventeenth to the twenty-third day after menstruation ceases.

During the first year of married life couples are liable to abuse the love sense by over-indulgence and thereby use up too much of their energy. This affects their health, especially that of the young wife, who finds herself always being tired and is unable to account for it. Her daily tasks become a drudgery, for she is too exhausted to have the strength to perform them. After the tasks finally are finished, she is too tired to don the afternoon dress, and so easily falls into untidy habits. This brings its train of results. The young husband, on his return from work, fails to find his wife the bright, attractive girl he married and gradually grows indifferent.

The relation of intercourse to conception is a problem that each husband and wife must settle for themselves. Some educators claim that only for the one is the other allowable, that the bearing and raising of children is the sole aim of married life. Naturally this is the fundamental end of the sex instinct. But in the present-day, practical married life it would be impossible to convince the majority that the impulse of sex gratification was given to them for this one purpose only.

The sense of well being and the increased capacity for work, that follows a moderate exercise of this function, tends to convince us that it has a beneficial effect upon the entire system if exercised moderately. As to what constitutes moderation or temperance depends upon the individual. What would be moderation to some would be excess to others. It may be taken as a general rule that the after-effects will indicate the amount. If the after-effects are irritability, extreme lassitude or a diminution of the love or respect for the other then there has been excess. If the after-effect is a sense of well-being so that the next day one feels more inclined to take up the duties of life, then it may be considered that moderation has been practiced. A certain amount of energy is consumed in any act and, as in our present age we need a great deal of energy to carry on our everyday business, in the majority of cases fresh vitality cannot be spared for an expenditure under several days or a week. Excess in anything tends to bring on premature old age, for the nervous force is expended faster than it is manufactured.

Frequently women seem to be endowed with an excess of energy which manifests itself in various forms. Besides this, the woman does not seem to have control of her nervous energy but wastes it in numerous ways. With many a woman the regularity and moderation attendant on a happy married life seems to have a regulating effect upon her whole nervous system, so that she becomes more calm and has greater control over her energies.

Wrong training or lack of training in matters pertaining to the relationship of the sexes and to the management of a home may be given as the cause of the majority of unhappy marriages.

There must be something wrong with our system of education when the aim of this education seems to be to prepare the girl for a temporary position in an office or store or for a gay social life; and when there is no preparation for the important work of home-making and the rearing of children. A girl would not be expected to run a complicated and delicate piece of machinery without having adequate instruction concerning the necessary care of it. But the girl is allowed to go blindly into marriage and is expected to manage her home and care for her children with practically no preparation. Nowadays we require experts for every position except that of motherhood, but we apparently do not consider that of enough importance to waste any time preparing for it. A man requires his gardener or office assistant to be trained, but the mother of his children need know nothing regarding the preparation for their coming. Too often her only preparation is that of making numerous clothes. She takes no measures to insure a healthy child.

If girls would make a study of home-making and motherhood and enter into marriage with a more definite realization of its obligations we would have fewer unhappy marriages and fewer divorce cases. Some women, owing to false education, wish to have all the advantages of marriage without assuming its cares. Such a woman expects a man to be willing to provide her with all the gifts of the gods, with all the luxuries of life, but in return is not willing to become the mother of his children nor to exert herself to make their mutual habitation a home and not merely a house--a place in which to eat and sleep.

A large part of the average woman's life is devoted to home-making and the rearing of children. Usually she is poorly prepared for this work. The early years of a girl's life are spent in the acquisition of a store of general knowledge, especially that derived from books and related to subjects generally considered necessary to "culture." During this period, her time is so occupied with her studies that her mother thinks it would be an imposition to ask her to do any housework, so the girl grows up without much knowledge of the care of a home. True, she often is enabled to do a few things. She learns to make cake and several varieties of candy and perhaps can fashion a collar that is the envy of her schoolmates. Sometimes she even helps her mother with the dishes or the dusting, but it is easier for the mother to take the responsibility of the housekeeping than it is to teach her daughter to do so, and besides her daughter always is so busy with school affairs. She has no time in which to learn the science of housekeeping.

After the completion of her course in the common or high school, a few months, sometimes, are devoted to the preparation for a certain line of work which is to occupy her time for a few years. Very few girls, except those who enter the professions, expect to continue their work after marriage and nearly all look forward to marriage. If we place a girl at a new occupation, for instance lace-making, and let her work out her own salvation, we would not be surprised if she disliked her work and was unable to accomplish any good results. But that is what we do in regard to home-making. A girl upon marriage is expected to know by instinct how to keep house, cook, and do the numerous other household duties; she is expected to know how to care for herself before the birth of her baby and how to care for the baby when it comes. Fortunately for the future generation this fact has come to the realization of many of our educators. During the last few years many schools have introduced into their curriculum, courses in domestic science, including the purchasing, preparation and serving of food. Very recently some of the more progressive schools have introduced courses in nursing and the care of young babies. Perhaps in a few years motherhood will take its proper place as the most important of all sciences.

CHAPTER VIII

EMBRYOLOGY--THE DEVELOPMENT OF LIFE

You remember I mentioned that at various times during the month an ovum or egg leaves the ovary and passes along the tube to the uterus. Here it remains if it is impregnated or fertilized by a union with the spermatozoon or male element. The whole body of the babe is developed from the ovum or female element after it has been fertilized by the spermatozoon or male element. The union usually takes place in the tube. The spermatozoon, after being deposited in the vagina, travels to the mouth of the womb, then up through the womb into one of the tubes. Here it meets the ovum and unites with it, then the impregnated ovum continues on its way to the uterus. It attaches itself to the lining of the womb by little thread-like filaments which it projects. The ovum then begins to grow, dividing itself into portions that go to make the different parts of the body. Before I continue, let me remind you that the ovum in the beginning is only about as large as the point of a pin, being about 1-125 of an inch in diameter, while the spermatozoon is so tiny it cannot be seen without the aid of a miscroscope. Therefore, it can be realized how much the ovum has to grow before it becomes a fully formed babe.

During the time the ovum is developing into the babe we speak of it first as the embryo, then the foetus. It takes about nine calendar months or ten lunar months before the foetus is fully developed and ready to be expelled from the womb. During the process of development the foetus resembles various animals. It seems it must pass through about the same stages of evolution that our primitive ancestors did.

By the end of the third week, the dividing has progressed so far that the body is quite well indicated. By the end of the seventh week the body and limbs are quite well defined. One peculiar thing is that, at this time, the foetus has a tail which disappears during the next two weeks. During the third month the foetus increases in size and weight so that by the end of the month the weight is four ounces and the length two and three-fourths inches. It now is not directly attached to the lining of the womb but is attached by means of the cord to the placenta or afterbirth which has been forming slowly. This placenta consists of fatty tissue surrounding a great many little blood vessels. The tiny blood vessels lie so close to the blood vessels of the lining of the womb that the blood passes from one to the other. To do this, it must pass through the walls of the blood vessels, as the vessels of the mother and those of the placenta are not directly united. The blood vessels of the placenta unite to form two veins and one artery which lie very close to each other and are surrounded by a membrane. These three blood vessels united together form what we call the cord. The other end of the cord is attached to the foetus so that the blood can flow back and forth between the foetus and placenta.

By the end of the third month the limbs have definite shape, the nails being almost perfectly formed. During the next month the sexual distinctions of the external organs become well marked.

By the last of the fifth month the weight has increased to one pound and the length to eight inches. Active foetal movements begin, that is, the foetus begins to move around and not lie quietly as before. This is what is usually spoken of as "feeling life," or as "quickening." There is life from the very beginning but during the first four or five months the foetus does not move about and so the mother does not "feel life." This has caused the erroneous idea that there is no life before the fifth month.

By the end of the sixth month the weight is two pounds and the length twelve inches. The eyebrows and eyelashes have begun to grow and the lobule of the ear is more characteristic.

By the end of the seventh month the weight is three pounds and the length fourteen inches. The surface of the body, which has appeared wrinkled, now appears more smooth owing to the increase of fat underneath.

By the end of the eighth month the weight is four to five pounds and the length twenty inches. The nails have grown to project beyond the finger tips.

Up to this time the body has been covered with a fine hair called lanugo. This now has begun to disappear and the skin becomes brighter and is covered with a white, cheesy material called the vernix caseosa. This almost entirely disappears during the next month, but frequently there are portions of it remaining on the body at the time of birth. The foetus is fully developed by the end of the ninth month. Then its average weight is six or seven pounds and the length twenty inches.

If we could look into the womb just before the time of labor we would find the foetus attached by the cord to the placenta and floating in a sac of water. This sac is formed partly of the placenta and partly of the membrane; the side of the placenta opposite to the child being attached to the womb. Just before labor the child takes a position with its head downward, its lower limbs flexed and its arms folded upon its breast. This allows it to come in the usual way, head first. But sometimes, for various reasons, it does not take this position and some part other than the head, for instance, the feet, may be born first.

Labor pains are caused by the contraction of the muscles of the womb in an effort to expel the foetus. The muscles, contracting, push the foetus downward to the mouth of the womb but push ahead of it a portion of the membrane enclosing some of the water. This is called the "bag of waters." As it presses against the mouth of the womb it causes it to dilate so as to allow the foetus to pass through into the vagina. The foetus, preceded by the bag of waters, then descends through the vagina or birth canal until it comes to the external opening of the vagina. This it must dilate before it can pass through it. The bag of waters should rupture normally while it is being pushed through the external opening. Sometimes the bag does not rupture directly in front of the descending head but further up along the side. Then a portion of the membrane may be over the face of the child when it is born. This is what is called being "born with a veil" or "born with a caul."

The bag of waters helps dilate the parts much easier than the foetus could do it alone. When the bag breaks the water lubricates the parts so as to make the passage of the child easier. When it breaks, as it sometimes does, at the beginning of labor we have what is termed a "dry labor." This usually is much slower than it would be otherwise. The majority of the cases of labor extend over a period of from twelve to twenty-four hours.

Sometimes the external opening of the vagina does not dilate enough to allow the passage of the child. As the head presses hard against the perineum it tears it. This tear should be repaired immediately after completion of labor.

When the baby is born it is fully formed but its lungs have never contained air. At the first cry the air rushes into the lungs and expands them. At birth there is a change in the circulation of the blood of the baby. Before this time, the blood has passed to and from the placenta through the cord but now this is stopped. Before birth there was an opening between the right and left sides of the heart but this closes during the first few days of the child's life. To assist in this closure, it is wise to keep the child on its right side for a few days. Rarely, this opening never closes and we have what is called a "blue baby," which seldom lives very long.

In a great many cases, painless childbirth could be a possibility by a little attention to diet, exercise and other hygienic measures during the last few months of pregnancy. Knowing this, it seems inconceivable that any woman would neglect to so fully inform herself on these matters that both she and her child could have all benefit of the investigations of science.

CHAPTER IX

ABORTIONS

Sometimes through an accident or on account of disease, the womb expels the foetus before it is fully developed. If this occurs before the end of the third month we call it an abortion; if it occurs between the third and seventh months we call it a miscarriage; while if it occurs after the seventh month but before the normal time of labor we call it a premature labor.

Formerly it was considered that there was no possibility of the child living if it were born before the seventh month. Now, by the aid of incubators, even those born at five months have a chance to live. By that time the body is fully formed, so the chief requirements are a steady temperature and proper care and food. Great care must be exercised, as a slight cooling of the air may result in the death of the babe.

Abortions are either accidental, criminal, or justifiable, that is, brought on to preserve the life of the mother. Accidental abortions may follow a sudden fall or a sudden shock, either mental or physical, to the mother. They may be due to some disease either of the mother or of the foetus. Of the diseases responsible for abortions the one with the largest percentage is syphilis. It is estimated that this disease is responsible for forty per cent. of accidental abortions and miscarriages. Whenever a physician has for a patient a woman who gives a history of having had several abortions without any apparent cause and all at about the same age of the foetus, he immediately becomes suspicious of syphilis either of the father or the mother. It is a peculiar fact with this disease that it may be transmitted to the offspring without the mother ever actually having the disease. This is an instance of "visiting the sins of the fathers upon the children unto the third and fourth generation." Many a weak frame owes its condition to a dissipated father, grandfather or even great-grandfather. It is possible, though, for a man or woman who has had this disease to have a healthy child if the disease has been properly treated.

Under some circumstances, especially with a deformed pelvis, if pregnancy were allowed to proceed normally it probably would result in the death of the mother. Then, it is considered justifiable for the physician in charge of the case to produce an abortion in order to save the life of the mother. Those cases are rare and such a procedure never is undertaken except in extreme cases.

Criminal abortions are those brought on simply because the woman does not desire to have a child. These often are produced by the woman herself by means of drugs that set up uterine contractions (labor pains) or by means of something introduced into the uterus. In either case it is a dangerous procedure. Infections may be carried into the uterus by means of whatever is introduced into it. This may set up an inflammation that may result in the death of the woman. It is a dangerous procedure to introduce anything into the womb. Some women are extremely foolish or reckless and use anything that may be handy. Sometimes grave harm results. Instances are on record of women who have punctured the walls of the womb by the use of hatpins or other sharp instruments. If an abortion is produced by either drugs or instruments there is danger that all the products of conception may not come away. If even a small portion remains in the uterus it may cause a hemorrhage or, becoming decomposed, produce a poison that may result in the death of the woman.

It would be impossible to estimate the number of abortions performed on unmarried girls, as well as married women, during one year by midwives, unscrupulous physicians and by many respected family physicians. We never hear of one of these except through the occasional one who is so unfortunate as to meet death. We cannot entirely blame the one who performs the abortion. Sometimes it is performed because of the sympathy of the physician. It is very hard to refuse some cases. Let me read you a letter to illustrate my meaning.

"I have just finished reading your article on 'Woman's Inhumanity to Woman' and wish to say that every word impresses the truth as read. My reason for writing you is because I am one of those who have sinned through love, with one I have known all my life only to find too late that he did not love me; and the sin is killing me. I do not want to bring into this world a little child to have no father. I am not bad at heart. My only hope is to get something that will bring me all right. If you are a doctor you can give me medicine that will help me miscarry this, as I have only missed two months. Nothing would please me more than to be the mother of a little one, but, oh, not one born without a name. Dear madam, if you can help me, or show me some way that my people cannot suspect me of this sin, for the love you bear all girls, help me. I am the only one at home to care for an aged father and one of the dearest brothers that ever lived. If he knew I had sinned as I have, it would break his heart. My God in heaven, help me! is my prayer, and through his love you can help me. I am almost desperate and before I will live and bear this sin I will take my own life, which will bar me from heaven and my angel mother's face. Be gracious, kind doctor, and help me. I will repay you if it takes the remainder of my life and give my solemn promise that I will sin no more. Erring through the love of a man is my only excuse and, oh, I am the one to bear the blame. He would be forgiven. I am so nervous and ruined in mind that I hardly can go about my duties and I cannot stand the strain much longer. Let me hear from you at once and please help me, for I know it can be done, but I am ignorant; I do not know what to get or what to do. It will be no sin to try to get all right and not bear a child, but in my thoughts it is something awful to have to have it. For the love of heaven help a heartbroken girl at once and before it is too late for me to regain my chance of heaven."

Now suppose you were a physician and that girl, instead of being a stranger, was a very dear friend who had come to you in your office, would you not be tempted to grant her wishes? That is the position in which every physician is placed a great many times. Some allow their sympathies to rule and so break the laws of the land. They allow their sympathies to overcome the moral truths that previously had been their guide. They commit a crime by taking a life, even though that life were not fully developed.

Many women have the false idea that there is no life before the fifth month and so think they are not destroying life if they have an abortion at the end of the first, the second or even the third month. This idea is entirely erroneous, for there is life from the very beginning and it is just as wrong to destroy life the first few months as it would be to do so later.

Aside from this moral reason there is a very important reason for not having abortions. You may regret it afterwards! Let me give you an instance. One of my friends, a charming young woman, was married several years ago. After her marriage she moved to a distant city and I did not see her for about four years. Then she returned and called to see me. During the course of our conversation I asked her if she had any children. Her reply in a very sad tone was, "No, I guess I did too much interfering at first, so now I cannot have any." Then she told me she had the idea she did not wish to have children for several years after she was married. So during the first year she had an abortion performed. Now for two years she had been wanting a baby but none came. That is the history of so many women. The regrets!

All women naturally desire to have children. If they do not, they are the victims of false ideas or of fear. Anything which is natural is the best, so usually a woman who bears children is much healthier than one who does not. Think of the women of your acquaintance and see if the mothers are not happier and healthier than the women who are childless.

CHAPTER X

MATERNAL IMPRESSIONS--HEREDITY

Every child has a right to be born well. An undesired child never should be brought into the world. An undesired child or a child of parents who are not in good bodily or mental condition comes into the world with an inheritance that perhaps never is overcome. How can we expect children of parents with criminal tendencies to become good citizens?

Children born in circumstances under which the expectant mother has been subjected to fright or to cruel treatment are handicapped in the very beginning of life's race. Maternal impressions from fright or physical violence undoubtedly are followed by the birth of individuals malformed and in many respects with altered minds. Although some biologists try to deny this, the coincidence is too widely observed to admit of doubt, although the precise manner in which the effect is produced has not been clearly demonstrated. Sufficient is known to make it of the utmost importance that, in the interest of her offspring, the expectant mother be not subjected to sudden or violent mechanical force or to any great nervous shock. Equally important is it that she should be surrounded by a harmonious environment in order to give the unborn child all possible benefit of such surroundings.

By many it is claimed that the mother's mental condition during this period will be reflected in the child both mentally and physically. For instance if the mother be calm, free from worry and happy in anticipation of the coming event, her offspring will have a sound nervous system, shown by a perfect digestion and an excellent disposition: while if the mother be irritable and unhappy her child is inclined to have various digestive ills, as well as to be cross and restless.

Great disturbances in the expectant mother's health also have their effect upon the child. The erroneous idea that there is no life before the third or fifth month allows many conscientious women to attempt measures that will cause the discharge of the products of conception. These measures not only are dangerous to the health or the life of the woman but, in the event of their proving unsuccessful, may result in the birth of a deformed or a mentally defective child.

Parents who have become degenerate from the immoderate use of alcohol or other stimulants or those who are afflicted with one of the black plagues furnish further examples of the birth of deficient offspring.

The question of heredity has received considerable attention during recent years. As a result, many of our pet theories have undergone a decided change. Many of the diseases which formerly were thought to be acquired through inheritance we now know to be contracted through lack of care or through association. The only inheritance is possibly a tendency to the disease or a decrease in the power of resistance. It is a law of pathology that the diseases of parents who suffer from certain serious chronic maladies create in the offspring a condition of defective life shown in malformations or in altered nutrition. The hereditary influence of most diseases is shown in the transmission to the child of a defective body shown by feebleness or a diminished power of resisting disease.

In tuberculosis and other diseases that once were considered hereditary, this influence is shown probably only in a predisposition to the disease which under favorable circumstances finds an easy condition of growth. The child does not actually inherit the disease and if placed in favorable surroundings will outgrow the tendency, will overcome the feeble vitality. But such a child if allowed to remain with its parent, to breathe the germs of disease cast off by the parent, readily contracts the disease. For the sake of the child it must be separated from its tubercular parent. It must be given fresh air and nourishing food.

There is one disease, though, that seems to be truly inherited: the worst of the black plagues, syphilis. This may be inherited from either parent, it frequently is inherited from the father even though the mother does not contract the disease. This inheritance seems to manifest itself chiefly in a disordered nutrition. Even during the first few months of development, this may be so effective as to destroy life. You remember, I mentioned this when I talked about abortions. If life is not destroyed, the nutritional processes may be so affected that the pregnancy will result in the birth of a defective child. These children, perhaps fortunately, usually die during the first few months of their lives. Seldom do they live to maturity. Many children who seem to have escaped this inherited trait really have not done so, but their inheritance is not recognized. Some people with defective generative organs owe this to a diseased parent. Others suffering from a chronic skin disorder, and many afflicted with epilepsy or some brain malformation could trace their inheritance to the same source. This disease seems truly to be an instance of "visiting the sins of the fathers upon the children unto the third and fourth generation."

There is no doubt that the general health of the child is affected by the health of the mother especially during the period when the child is nourished from the mother's blood. Attention to such matters as diet, sleep and exercise certainly has a great influence upon the constitution of the unborn child. The best heritage a mother can give her child is a strong constitution, and in order to do this she must make motherhood a science.

CHAPTER XI

CHILDLESS HOMES AND REAL HOMES--CAUSES OF STERILITY

Whatever may be the motive that causes men and women to enter into matrimony, the social reason is the perpetuation of the human race. Herbert Spencer says, "The welfare of the family underlies the welfare of society." Therefore those who marry for convenience or with the avowed intention of not assuming the obligations of parenthood have not the welfare of the human race at heart and are a menace to society in its highest form.

Childless homes are not the happy homes, anyhow! Their occupants usually are dissatisfied; the women are nervous, irritable and unhappy; the men are seeking happiness elsewhere. The homes childless from choice should receive our condemnation, but the homes childless from necessity should receive our commiseration. The latter are much more prevalent than many of our race suicide agitators would admit. These are too prone to blame the woman for what is not her choice. We hear so much about the higher education of women promoting race suicide. A recent investigation carried on by a well-known magazine has proven that such is not the case. The college girls and the professional women desire children much more than do the factory girls. But these college girls realize that quality is as necessary as quantity. They do not desire to bring into the world weak, puny offspring. These college girls are beginning to make motherhood a science. What the results will be we can only anticipate.

A normal woman, who has not become imbued with false ideas and fear, desires children. She realizes that motherhood, if rightly carried out, is a privilege and not a curse; it is the woman who has been falsely educated who dreads motherhood. This morning I received a letter which shows the prevailing attitude of many girls. The writer says:

"I am twenty-two years of age but strange to say I am ignorant as far as knowledge about the origin of life, etc., is concerned. I am a business girl, drawing a good salary, and have many gentleman and lady friends. I am the oldest child of a large family of moderate means and have been brought up under Christian principles and possess a goodly amount of common sense. I long have been anxious in regard to this important subject but never have asked anyone for advice, shuddering to do so, feeling that if I had a chance to ask a lady with knowledge, as a nurse or some such person, I would do so. But to tell the truth, I did not care to find out such things, but I realize the fact that I must know in order to guard myself; for that is something no one can do for me at a critical moment. I have no less than three gentleman admirers, but I have no desire to be a married woman for a long time to come, but I feel that I must be armed with the knowledge of right and wrong. I shudder on account of fear to think of becoming a mother. I hear so much of woman's pains and aches and the such, that I often think I would prefer to remain single all my life, although I am perfectly healthy and a happy, cheerful girl. My mother is, and always will be, too busy to tell me about such matters, although I had a right to know long ago. As you say, an ignorant, innocent girl would be guilty before the world if something wrong should happen to her and in most cases it is not her fault. Can you give me the desired information or can you recommend some good book? If so, I assure you that your efforts will be greatly appreciated."

This letter certainly indicates that the writer has a good amount of common sense. The trouble is she has become over-impressed with the possibilities of pain, and never has been told the wonderful truths that would overcome this fear. If love is the greatest thing in the world, fear and its companion, worry, certainly are the greatest curses of humanity. And the most pitiful part is that this fear and worry usually result from ignorance which a little instruction at the right time could dispel so easily. It is the unknown things that we fear. When any trouble actually comes we find strength enough to meet it, and, anyway, it usually is not half as bad in the reality as in the prospect. Young girls hear so much about the pains of childbirth that this fear overshadows the natural longings for motherhood. It is not until motherhood is an actual fact that they realize the happiness is worth all the cost.

But this fear is not what actually makes many childless homes. They often are unpremeditated. A large percentage of the sterility in the world is due to the results of indiscretions that are the outcome of ignorance. One great factor in childless homes is the prevalence of the black plagues. It is estimated that forty-five per cent. of sterile marriages are due to that seemingly mild disease which is regarded as no worse than a cold and which has been contracted either by the man or the woman. This disease does not disqualify the woman alone, as was formerly thought, for recent investigations have proven that twenty-five per cent. of the sterile marriages are due to sterility of the male. Oh, the innumerable women who have submitted to unpleasant treatments and even operations in the hope of overcoming sterility when all the time the fault was elsewhere! The microscope has proven that even though a man may seemingly be healthy and capable of sustaining the marriage relation, yet his efforts are valueless; for the spermatozoa, the life-giving element, are dead, due usually to an inflammation which accompanied an attack of this seemingly mild disease,-- gonorrhoea.

This disease is responsible for many of the one child marriages. How often we see a family with only one child, this child born during the first year of married life, then there are no more pregnancies. The woman probably has contracted a disease from her husband and, during the period immediately following the birth of her baby when the entire generative system is in a condition to easily become inflamed, the tubes have become closed. Another pregnancy is very unlikely.

Another factor in sterility is abortions. So many times we hear a young married woman say, "I do not want a child the first year, but after that I would like one." In order to carry out her desires it is not uncommon for an abortion to be performed during the first few months. In many cases an inflammation follows this interference and the tubes become closed permanently. Then when the woman is ready to have a child it is impossible. Girls about to enter marriage should be cognizant of this possibility and not take any risks, for few women would do anything voluntarily that would condemn them to childless lives.

CHAPTER XII

PREVENTION OF PREGNANCY

This morning I received a letter which says in part, "I am a young school teacher and do not know lots I should, but will come to you for advice. Now I am engaged to the dearest boy in the world. I will do my best to be a good wife and do my duty. But my health is not so very good and I want to put off motherhood for awhile. Will you kindly tell me some remedy that will keep me from becoming pregnant? I have long wanted to ask someone but always was afraid. Mother never tells me anything."

This is the type of question that is asked every physician many times. Those who do not ask, wish to--and blame physicians for not telling the things they want to know. What is my answer to such a question? Just this:

There is in effect a federal statute making it a felony punishable by $5,000 fine and five years at hard labor to impart any information whatever relating to the preventing of conception. The information may concern a thing, an instrument, or it need not be any material substance at all--only a "method." I obey that law as I am not foolhardy enough to walk into absolute danger.

Every day we see examples of heart-breaking misery caused by lack of knowledge of the proper means of prevention. The limitation of the number of offspring has become an important problem to be considered. There are thousands of families that would be perfectly happy if the number of offspring could be limited. There are thousands of young men who would be glad to get married but are afraid to do so for fear of having a family larger than they could supply with the necessities of life. These same young men, because they are not married, frequent questionable houses and often contract one or more of the venereal diseases.

There are thousands of women who have become semi-invalids because of a too prolific offspring. The babies came so fast the mother had no opportunity to regain her health and strength. There are other thousands of women who are made invalids because of attempts at abortion, or have been driven into early graves by these attempts, while some have actually killed themselves.

There are thousands of children half starved because their parents are unable to supply them the necessities of life. There are other thousands of children below par mentally and physically because of the fact that the mother was weak from too frequent child-bearing. There are other thousands of children born of syphilitic, tubercular or epileptic parents who never should have been born at all because they came into life so handicapped and had to fight against such severe odds that they, after a brief struggle, met an early death. There are children brought into this world amidst cursing who never hear much else.

We find it necessary to regulate the parentage of our domestic animals in order to insure a good race. But children can come by chance. The most degraded of men is allowed to beget children of his kind. There is small chance for race improvement under such conditions. The same laws hold true as to the future generation of humans as are true of animals or plants.

Human beings are not mere animals and they should be allowed to decide how many children they should have. Furthermore, the present laws do not attain their object. We all pretend to obey the laws but everyone knows that in every city there are many women, and men also, who make an excellent income from performing abortions. I would venture to say that in Chicago alone there is at least one abortion performed every hour--and Chicago is not so very different from other parts of the country in this respect. The ways and means to prevent pregnancy are sold and are bringing a rich reward to their manufacturers. But the advertisements are so carefully worded that the law is not violated. But the interested understand. If the manufacturer or his agent were accused of selling anything to prevent pregnancy, he would simulate great surprise and possible indignation. He doing such a thing! Impossible! Why, he is selling a simple hygienic device or drug used in the treatment of certain diseases.

If we have laws, let us obey them; but if we do not intend to obey them, let us stop being hypocrites and remove them from the statutes. If the law remains let us make it far-reaching enough to include those who now are so flagrantly violating it. But if means for the prevention of pregnancy are necessary to the health and happiness of the human race, let us change the laws so we can have the best of these preventives and allow reputable physicians to give whatever information they can to prevent this wholesale misuse of a law by the unscrupulous,--the law-breakers.

A recent investigation carried on by one magazine proved that the knowledge of how to prevent conception would not mean race suicide, as some fear. As reported in this magazine, the college girls and professional women who no doubt had given these subjects careful consideration, desired children more than did those whose experience had been a poor home and a large family. The average number of children desired by the well-informed woman was four. That would not mean race-suicide! It would mean that children were given a fair start in life by being desired and planned for before their conception. Every true woman desires a home and children but she does not wish to be driven into motherhood. Every true man desires a family but he does not feel justified in bringing children into the world to be half starved and with no advantages of education.

What is the solution of the problem?

CHAPTER XIII

SOME OF THE CAUSES OF DIVORCE

Until our marriage laws are so adjusted that there are no unequal marriages, the question of divorce always will be eminent. The ever present agitation about uniform divorce laws and the divorce problem cannot be settled until there are more stringent marriage laws. Trying to settle the divorce question without first settling the marriage question is like trying to keep chickens in a small yard surrounded by enticing fields without first constructing an adequate fence.

Divorce is the concession of society to its inability to solve the marriage problem. Anyone can get married! Mere children can meet on a pleasure excursion and in a moment of fun or infatuation walk over to a justice of the peace and be married. In some states not even a license is necessary. A large proportion of the marriages in the world are consummated without a proper consideration on the part of either bride or groom as to the responsibilities of the marriage state. Many of the marriages are made simply as a matter of convenience--in order to inherit property, for social position or in a spirit of pique. Such marriages are not natural marriages and are in violation of the right spirit of the law of marriage. The much quoted saying, "What God hath joined together, let no man put asunder," surely does not apply to these marriages; for that very admission would be a condemnation of the wisdom of God. He surely never would give his sanction to many of the marriages contracted in a spirit of lust or of greed.

It is as impossible to keep mismated people together as it is to keep chemical incompatibles together. No chemist would try to keep chlorate of potash and sulphur together even if they did, by some accident, happen to be in the same locality. It is just as impossible to keep two incompatible people together and not expect an explosion. The law may keep such people legally bound, but it cannot keep them so mentally or physically. A prominent reformer is reported to have said that fully one-third of the married population of New York City is unfaithful to the physical obligation. And New York is not so very different from other parts of the country. Many who are not physically disloyal are mentally so. The no-divorce law will not prevent this condition of affairs. Whites and blacks cannot marry legally in the South and yet in some of the Southern states which have a no-divorce system a large proportion of the colored population is mulatto.

Nature's laws tend to provide an indissoluble union, but divorce represents the protest of the individual against the inharmonious relations he ignorantly or thoughtlessly has assumed.

Even those who are the loudest in their condemnation of divorce could not sanction marriage under certain conditions. I wonder if these people know that many of the divorces that are granted under the head of cruelty really are granted because one of the parties has contracted one of the loathsome black plagues. No humane person could condemn a woman for refusing to live with a man and take the almost certain risk of contracting a disease that would mean her death or mutilation, or for refusing to bear children that would come into the world an object of disgust and horror or which would die before being born. Some of these reformers say, "Let her live separately from him but not marry again." That would be condemning an innocent woman to a childless life because she had been so unfortunate as to become bound to a dissipated man.

Another underlying but often unknown factor in many of the divorce cases is sterility. In some states the law says this is a just cause for divorce, because the future of the nation depends on the production of children. Because a woman, in her ignorance, has married a man who is incapable of producing healthy offspring, due to his having "sown his wild oats," should not be a reason why she should be condemned to forego the pleasures of motherhood. Because a man has married a woman who is sterile or who selfishly refuses to bear children should not be a reason why he should be denied an heir.

Again, it is unfair to the future generation to compel mismated couples to live together. Children brought into the world under such conditions are bequeathed a heritage that will have a demoralizing effect upon their whole after life. Children, who every day hear quarrels and strife between those they should honor, lose something of the beauty of life; they become hardened and quarrelsome. Of course these divorces must not be granted promiscuously; for in bringing children into the world, parents assume an obligation that cannot be neglected. In considering a separation, the parents' first thought should be, "What is best for my children?" The duty to the children should be settled first. Then the question comes, "What is my duty to my wife or my husband?" for the act of making any contract imposes certain obligations. The individual circumstances must settle what these obligations are. Last comes the question, "What is my duty to myself? I was placed in this world to make the best use of my life. Am I doing it or is it impossible to do so unless I change my environment and associates?" The conscience of the individual should be the guide now.

Were there more frankness and sincerity in discussing the problems and conditions of married life before marriage much unhappiness would be avoided and there would be fewer divorces; for many engaged people would thus discover they were mismated before the marriage ceremony. To reach a complete understanding is the main purpose of the engagement period. Marriage is not a lottery nor a game of chance to the man and woman entering it with a knowledge of sex relations and with absolute mutual honesty.

CHAPTER XIV

THE NEED OF EARLY INSTRUCTION OF GIRLS

Dr. Charles W. Eliot, former president of Harvard University, recently said:

"The subject of reproduction and sexual hygiene should be more generally presented to young people by parents and teachers. I am convinced that the policy of silence has failed disastrously."

That you may understand how widely spread is this desire on the part of women for a better knowledge of themselves and of those things so vitally important to the welfare of the future generation, I shall quote a few extracts from letters I have received from women in various parts of the country. These letters, too, will serve to show the woeful ignorance along these lines among even the well educated women, and also the need for some systematic instruction.

A very intelligent girl from South Dakota writes this heart story: "My mother died when I was a babe. After her death I was sent out among strangers. While away from home and before I was six years old a young fellow about fifteen years old possessed me and threatened to do something terrible to me if I told. I did not dare tell. Luckily I was taken home at that time, as I now had a step-mother. But still more horrible, it also happened that I had immoral relations with my brother. When I found out that this was the way people got babies, I wished I could get one. I was not very old before I understood that this was a wrong and a shame and acted accordingly. My parents never mentioned things of this nature to me. How much better it would have been if they had done so when we were real young. How many things were spoken of by schoolmates and told in the dirtiest possible way and things also were said that I now know were entirely wrong."

I cannot impress upon you too strongly the need of early talks with young children on these matters. As soon as they enter school at the age of six and even before this, in some cases, they are bound to hear these things from their playmates. Usually the information is thrust upon the child in a very vulgar manner, or entirely wrong impressions are given. The very secrecy that always has surrounded these subjects makes them an object of interest to children. The functions of the generative organs are just as natural a process as the process of digestion. We make no secret of the process of digestion, and children do not manifest any morbid curiosity regarding it. If we would discuss the functions of the generative organs in just as natural a way, many of our great problems would right themselves.

A woman in one of the western states writes, "Once I had a heated argument upon that subject with another woman. She always had lived in a small community. In her opinion all city girls were morally depraved. She had two daughters of her own. Both girls gave birth to babies at the age of fourteen and sixteen years. It transpired later that these girls first began the evil practice at school. And I will state here, regardless of contradiction, that the village school is often the breeder of immoral characters among both boys and girls.

"In a small farming community of California containing about forty children of school age, it was discovered that immoral practices had been carried on for years among the older children. One little girl, being new to the school and also being in the habit of telling her mother everything, repeated some of the sights she had seen during the recess and noon hours, and also some of the conversation she had heard among the children. The mother, being horrified at the child's revelations and knowing the child must have some foundation for her stories, told a friend about it. This woman told some of her friends who were the mothers of the children the little girl had named to her mother. Of course, the children were questioned and denied all knowledge of things the child had mentioned. The mothers were indignant that their children should be accused of anything like that. They unquestionably believed the denial, making no effort to find out if there might be any truth in the report. That mother and her little one were 'sent to Coventry' with a vengeance. Later some of these mothers had cause to repent of their carelessness in having neglected or disregarded the warning. They found to their sorrow that the little girl was not telling an untruth, after all.

"The trouble with the mother in the small community is that she judges her children by her own past. She, perhaps, had an entirely different environment from that of her children and because she came out all right, naturally sees no use in bothering about talking to her girls. 'They will learn these things soon enough,' she says when the subject is mentioned. That they either already have learned them or may be learning them in a manner of which she would be the last to approve, she does not take into consideration. An attempt to warn such a mother often is misunderstood."

That young women realize their need and are anxious for any help is shown by these letters. From New York a girl writes, "I am twenty-two years of age and as yet know nothing about the mysteries of life, and I am beginning to worry about it as I am keeping company with a young man and expect to become engaged to him. I know nothing of what is expected of me when I get married and I know there are a number of girls just like me and that they are worried, too."

From a girl in Seattle came this letter, "No one ever told me about this wonderful body of ours and that God made it in his likeness for his glorification. When I asked where the babies came from, I was told the doctor brought them in his case. One day I saw a boy and girl about eight years of age doing wrong, and thought nothing of it when my brother, who was fourteen while I was six, proposed that we do likewise. This was kept up until I was somewhere between eleven and thirteen, when I was converted and it occurred to me that this was not the right thing to do, but I never dreamed that I would suffer so these ten years, as I am twenty-three now. Only in the last few years I have learned how God made these organs for the marriage relation only and how life was formed. I would go to my mother for this information but I know it would break her heart and I am afraid she could not tell me what I want to know. I would not write this but I am deeply in love with a Christian man, and I could not marry anyone until I know about this matter. I often have made a vow I never would marry anyone, but this love came to me before I could help myself, and as he told me of his love I would not allow myself to let him know I care as much as I do. Kindly tell me if anyone who has abused her organs while so young could make a good wife or become a mother, and can these marks of sin be removed?"

Another young girl writes, "It is just as you say, ignorance is the root of evil in many cases such as mine. I have come to you for help, information and advice. I have taken that fatal mis-step you write about, but no one knows it besides myself and this man. He dare not speak of this. He is very wealthy and influential. After reading your article I found that you were the one to go to and make a confession. I never have been warned or told of these dangers and now it is too late. I am a young girl, eighteen years old, and have a lot of men friends because I am considered attractive, but none of them have ever said one word out of the way to me except this one and I yielded to the tempter. I know I have done wrong, and now am trying to atone for it by being awfully good. Now, what I want to know and want you to tell me is this, 'Can I ever marry a decent, respectable man without him knowing of this affair?' There is a young man very much devoted to me (and I can assure you it is mutual) who several times has asked me to marry him. I am afraid to give him an answer. I cannot ask anyone else this question for the simple reason that I am not sure whether they will tell me the truth or whether they really know."

Both these girls were fortunate that they did not have any serious consequences from their mis-step. Too many girls make only one mis-step and as a result become pregnant or else contract one of the black plagues. This week I have received several such letters. Laying aside all moral points, it is too much risk for any girl to run.

Unfortunately a great many girls in their ignorance do make a mis-step. That is no reason why they should not marry. We must take into consideration the fact that the young man in question probably has made several of these mis-steps. He should not expect his prospective wife to be any stronger to resist temptation than he has been. If this were an ideal world, all men, as well as all women, would be pure, but until the millennium comes we must take things as they are, and proceed from that standpoint. But because a girl has erred through ignorance is no reason why she should be doomed to everlasting punishment in the shape of social ostracism or being denied the happiness of having a home and children.

These are only a few of the many letters I have received, but they serve to show the great need of early instruction of girls on these much neglected subjects. Every girl, soon after she enters school if not before, learns where babies come from. She too often is led by older children, both boys and girls, to do things she may regret later. It has been said that "sin is but ignorance." This is true in the great majority of cases of immoral practices among girls as well as among boys. The remedy for these sins, then, is to do away with the ignorance by proper instruction of children. Children are reasonable beings and if they understood the why would not do wrong.

If girls go wrong through ignorance the parents are to blame; for at the present time there is no excuse for a parent not giving the necessary instruction. If, on account of her own lack of knowledge, the mother feels incapable of instructing her daughter, there are others ready and willing to aid her; also, there are books especially prepared for her help, which will definitely point the way.

CHAPTER XV

WHY GIRLS GO ASTRAY

Not long ago an estimable young woman in speaking of the unfortunate girls in the world said, "I cannot see how any refined girl could get into trouble. I cannot conceive of any circumstances which would permit any self-respecting girl to allow the familiarities necessary for such a condition." That is the attitude assumed by many intelligent women. Because they grew up in an environment without temptations, because they had no unsatisfied longings to be loved or to be popular, they are incapable of understanding these feelings in any other person.

In every girl there is an inborn longing to be loved and to have a home of her own. It is a misunderstanding of this sense that is responsible for the wrecked lives of many girls. In too many homes there is no expression of the love sense. Frequently I have heard girls remark, "Why, I never think of kissing my parents except, perhaps, when they or I go away." In too many homes the only mention that is made of love is that made in a bantering manner. A child has the right idea of love. She loves everyone and is free in the expression of this love. As she grows older she obtains wrong ideas of love and she too often obtains these wrong ideas in her own home and from her own parents who instill false ideas of love when indulging their habit of "teasing." Frequently we hear parents talking about the small daughter's "beau." The child feels pent-up emotions of love and, as there is no outlet at home in a natural way, she acquires the idea that these emotions should be spent in a childish love affair.

In a recent address Professor Marx Lubine of the University of Berlin said, "Motherhood, in all stages of civilization, has been strangely ignorant of the fact that girls have as powerful a battery of emotions as boys. It is my experience that a major portion of mothers understand their sons better than their daughters. Why? The daughters are not given credit for a power of emotion the sons are capable of. Yet, naturally, in my long experience with both sexes, I have no hesitation in saying that the emotions of a pure girl are usually deeper, more lasting, than those of a boy, and that if we are to have a great improvement in womanhood it must come through a recognition of this fact."

It is strange but mothers seem to be blind to, or ignorant of the emotions that are seething back of the clear eyes of their daughters. The emotions of the girl have not been studied sufficiently. We expect a boy to do things which serve as an outlet to his pent-up emotions but we expect a girl to go on in a calm, uneventful manner with no outlet for the overflow of emotions. Blessed are the "Tomboys." I would there were more of them. It is a fact that the girl who runs, plays, climbs trees and is given to outdoor sports generally during the early part of her life develops into the truest woman. She has an outlet for her energies. Her time is fully occupied with those things that promote health. She has no time nor desires for those things that show a perverted taste. Such a girl seldom becomes a victim of self-abuse. She is not inclined to romantic love affairs. It is her sister who sits and sews who has time and inclination for indulging in morbid longings and who becomes the victim of pernicious habits.

Curiosity is one of the prominent characteristics of both sexes. With the boy this is satisfied without much pretence at secrecy. False modesty prevents the girl from openly obtaining the desired information. She obtains it secretly from her companions. Mothers do not give their daughters credit for the instinct that compels the satisfaction of their curiosity. Sometime during her life, nearly every mother is surprised and shocked at the knowledge displayed by her daughter. She finds that owing to her silence and neglect of opportunities her daughter has obtained definite if entirely wrong ideas of sexual matters.

In other matters, too, the policy of silence or of arbitrarily forbidding the daughter to indulge in certain pleasures, coupled with the natural curiosity of the girl, tends to develop in her the habit of deceitfulness. If she is forbidden some harmless amusements she very frequently learns these diversions at the homes of her friends. The mother was brought up in one generation, the daughter in another; what was considered wrong in the first generation is looked upon in an entirely different manner now. Many mothers seem to be unable to realize this. They were brought up in a puritanical environment. The puritan fathers forbade all indulgence in mirth and happiness. Their ideas of the perfect life were to wear a stern, unsmiling countenance and do those things that were unpleasant. If anything was uncongenial, then it was their duty to overcome their inclinations. These puritans expected to develop by repression. We have changed our ideas radically since then, but some of the puritanical ideas still cling to us in our treatment of children. To develop the child's character she must be made to do the things she does not want to do and to refrain from the things she most desires. Is it right?

We are most interested in those things that belong to us individually or in which we have some share. If we wish a girl to remain at home then we must see that she is interested in that home. The way to do this is to make her feel that the home belongs to her in part and that some portions of it are entirely hers. The majority of girls feel no real interest in their homes. They are made to feel that it is their parents' home and that they are only assistants. A girl to be interested in her home must have some definite room that is hers alone and in which she is allowed to exercise her individual tastes. She must have a place in which she can entertain her friends without the feeling that whatever she does and says is to be criticised afterwards. She should be assigned to certain tasks and held responsible for them. She must have a certain definite allowance out of which she is to buy certain things, otherwise her desire for independence will arise and cause her to leave home. The majority of girls have no income of their own. Perhaps their desires are all fulfilled by an indulgent parent and yet the girls resent the feeling of dependence.

Girls are naturally just as ambitious as boys, and they need good, honest work to keep them healthy and their minds occupied. If a girl displays an interest in a certain line of work this interest must be encouraged. Usually it is not. The girl is taught, either consciously or unconsciously, that whatever occupation she takes up will be only temporary, that to become engrossed in her work would mean no marriage. Girls cannot do good work under such conditions.

CHAPTER XVI

SELF-ABUSE

In one of my articles for one of the leading women's magazines I spoke of mental self-abuse. This brought me so many inquiries regarding both mental and physical self-abuse that I feel impelled to explain them to you.

To abuse means to use wrongly, or to injure. We have talked about the uses of the female organs and also about the care of them. Sometimes, I have watched children rub their eyes until they were quite red and inflamed. I have seen children, thoughtlessly, stick pins and hairpins in their ears and I even have had to remove a bean which a thoughtless child had pushed up its nose. All these things did more or less harm to the parts. In the same way, some girls play with their external generative organs and even put things up in the vagina. Sometimes they injure these organs greatly, and sometimes there is a more general and serious effect. You know the nerves of the body all are very closely connected like telegraph wires so that an irritation to one part will sometimes be telegraphed to another entirely different part and cause the nerves of that part to be irritated. When you have a toothache your whole face and head and even your arms ache. That is because the nerves are irritated. In the same way if one irritates the nerves of the female organs, the whole body may be affected; only in this case it is more serious than with the toothache; for these female organs are more abundantly supplied with nerves.

One who is guilty of such an unnatural practice as to deliberately irritate any portion of her body, especially the very important generative organs, always secretly despises herself. If persisted in, the results of this vice are a ruined nervous system and a weakened character. The victim realizes she is doing a disgraceful thing and seldom acknowledges her habit even to her physician.

If one has become a victim of such a habit she should determine to stop it immediately and then take measures to restore her nervous system to its original state. It never is too late to commence treatment. It is the continued practice and the mental dwelling on the acts that does the harm, not the few acts thoughtlessly performed. Of course the longer the habit has continued, the more firmly it is fixed and the harder to break.

The treatment is first to absolutely stop the practice, then fill your mind with other thoughts. Take considerable physical exercise in the open air. Sleep on a hard bed in a well-ventilated room. Eat plain, nourishing food without spices and stimulants. Take up some work or play that will interest you and that will keep your mind occupied. Live in the open air as much as possible. If you find yourself desiring to do these harmful things, go immediately and busy your mind and hands with something else and the desire will pass soon. In young children this habit often has its origin in some irritation of the external organs, as a hooded clitoris. So before taking severe measures to break the habit, it is wise to have the child examined for such a condition.

Now as to mental self-abuse, perhaps I can make my meaning more clear by again quoting from some of my letters. A young woman from South Carolina wrote me, "A few years ago I taught school and one of my pupils, perfectly innocent of the grave results that would befall her, committed three outrages upon herself, what is known in the medical world as masturbation or self-abuse. The girl, as I know, was chaste and a sweeter, nicer, brighter pupil I never taught. But she had the misfortune to commit these abuses upon herself in all innocence and felt no discomfort or ill health in any way until about three months afterward. Then she began to lose interest in her work, to fall away in her grades, in fact to take very little interest in anything. In this condition she came to me and told me everything. Since then she has felt no physical pain whatever, but her mind, though not really gone, is visibly affected. In this way, she is constantly in dread lest something dreadful will happen, feels as if a cloud were hanging over her, is not capable of doing any mental work. At times, has a horror of being shut up in any place, memory is poor, places and positions change, that is, a place moves to some other position, for instance, the right side of the street very often is in the opposite direction. To sum it all up, she constantly is miserable. So far as being insane is concerned, she is not that. She is perfectly conscious of her condition. She feels well physically and appears to be so mentally, but says there is just a befogged sensation in her head which gets no better nor worse, yet it is there. The feeling came upon her very suddenly one morning in the spring after the abuses had taken place in January and then it all flashed over her the awful consequences of her innocent practices. Oh! what would she not have given to be her old self again! If she only had known the awful result, her mind sacrificed for a practice in which she indulged through ignorance and for experiment, never dreaming the baneful effect it would have on her mind. Now, this girl has gone on this way for the past eight years getting no worse nor any better. Seemingly, she is the same but she suffers untold miseries when alone, conscious that her mind is hazy and not capable of enjoying books, society of others or anything that interests young girls. Yet nobody ever would detect that she is not feeling well. She told me all this in confidence and as the case puzzles me, I write you feeling that perhaps you would advise me in some way the treatment necessary to cure her. She is and has been perfectly moral since the fateful abuses upon herself and I do not understand why her mind does not return to its normal condition."

I do! She will not give her mind a chance to get well. She constantly is abusing it by dwelling on things that should have been forgotten long ago. No one goes through life without making some mistakes. Everyone has burned his finger many times. And yet he does not keep worrying about it and wondering if it will have some dangerous after-effect. Of course, if he deliberately burned his finger time and time again, it might remain injured permanently. But if he, ignorantly or accidentally, has burned it once or several times, he stops his careless ways, allows Nature to restore the injured portion, and then forgets there ever was an injury. It is the same with self-abuse, many children do things like this thoughtlessly. But when a girl learns she is injuring herself, she should stop the practice and allow Nature to repair the wound. Then forget all about it. Do not worry, above all things. Go ahead and fill your mind with work.

There are many women in this world who are abusing themselves by worrying over something that has occurred in the past. Whatever is in the past cannot be undone. All we can do is to profit by our experience and turn the energies, that would be wasted by worrying, to some good use. Whenever thoughts of the past or desires for the wrong things disturb you, crowd these worry thoughts and desires out of your mind by putting in it good thoughts. Deliberately fill your mind and hands so full of other things that there will be no room for these unwholesome pests. Worry does more harm than smallpox ever did!

This dwelling on past mistakes is only one of several methods of mental self-abuse. Another way some abuse themselves is by continuing the association with those who excite or irritate them. If in your work or social life you find that a certain person has an effect upon you that is not wholesome, that when you are in the company of that individual you are incapable of doing your best, then it is time to make a change. Keep away from that individual until such a time as you are strong enough to resist his influence. Choose your friends from among those who stimulate you mentally. If you stop to think, you must admit that you accomplish more and better work when in the presence of certain people. Those are the ones whose companionship you should seek.

There are people living together or working together who are a continual source of irritation to each other. It is just as impossible for such people to work in harmony as it is for two incompatible chemicals, as nitrogen and iodine. We do not try to over-ride the laws of Nature by trying to force these chemicals to stay together. It is just as impossible to force certain incompatible people to be harmonious. If society or business throws two such people together it would be wise for one to make a change before there is an explosion. It is impossible for any person to do good work in an atmosphere of irritation.

Another element in mental self-abuse is longing for the unattainable. Sometimes a person sets her mind on a certain thing. If that goal is an honorable one, she should make every effort to attain it but if circumstances over which she has no control make that goal impossible of attainment she should turn her thoughts in another direction. But that is what many people do not do. If they cannot have just what they want they sit and bemoan their fate and give up trying for other goals. Such a person should choose a line of work or play that is especially interesting to her and bend her energies in that direction. She will be surprised how soon she will lose her intense interest in her former longed-for goal.

Lack of self-confidence is an evidence of mental self-abuse. A person who has no confidence in herself cannot expect others to have. One who keeps herself in the attitude of Uriah Heap, who continually asserts, "I am a poor worm, I am unworthy of the blessings of life, I cannot expect great reward," must expect to be taken at her word. In this age a man (or woman) is valued, in a large measure, by the estimate he sets upon himself. Honors are not thrust upon a man unless he shows the self-confidence which commands confidence. Bacon said, "Some are born great, some achieve greatness and some have greatness thrust upon them." But those of the last class are very few. Our enemies are willing to thrust upon us scandal and humiliation whenever there is a possible chance, but our friends are very slow in thrusting honors upon us. If a person wants anything in this world he must first convince himself of his ability to attain that goal, then he may be able to convince others. It is the man with confidence in himself who wins the day.

After one has decided upon his goal he should keep that goal always before him as the pillar of fire before the seekers for the promised land. All our thoughts should be in that direction. Every wish or thought we send out reaches someone and in time may bring us what we wish. "By faith ye can accomplish all things."

There is an explanation of "Who answers prayer" which describes a mother kneeling by the bedside of her sick baby, and praying faithfully that her baby might be restored to health. In a vision the author sees these prayer thoughts radiating from the mother like invisible telegraph wires, along which the message is carried to various parts of the city. One wire reaches the home of a minister who, although willing, feels his inability to answer. Another wire reaches the home of a wealthy banker but he, too, is powerless to help. The next wire is connected with the home of a prominent lawyer famous for his ability to win cases for the needy, but in this case he cannot win, for Death is more powerful than he. But a fourth wire reaches a physician who has just retired from a hard day's fight with his enemy--disease. The physician awakens, grasps the message and immediately arises, dresses and hastens to the home of the poor woman. In a short time the little one's spasms are relieved and the doctor gives a sigh of relief, as he says to the anxious mother, "The crisis is past, your baby will live." The mother's prayer has been answered.

Every thought we entertain is being sent out along these invisible wires and eventually will reach someone who responds to it. If we send out worry thoughts or thoughts of self-depreciation we must expect others to receive the message as we send it. So if we want to make the most of our lives we continually must send out only thoughts that we wish others to receive. We must value ourselves if we expect others to value us!

Too much introspection and concern for self is often the cause of nervous conditions that produce worry and ill-health. The best cure is the cultivation of complete unselfishness. To be interested in the happiness of others is the surest road to happiness for one's self;--if you get feeling tired of yourself make a visit to some congenial friend, and there forget self and your troubles. "It is more blessed to give than receive" is a truth that all serene and great souls recognize and practice throughout their lives.

CHAPTER XVII

EFFECTS OF IMMORAL LIFE

Some time ago, the general public was shocked by a newspaper story of the life led by many girl clerks in the department stores of a large city. It seems a young girl from the country applied for a position in one of the stores, but upon hearing of the small wages paid, said, "How can I live on that? It would not provide even the most meager of board and the smallest room." The employer asked in reply, "But have you not a gentleman friend?" That reply, repeated to a social worker, started an investigation which resulted in startling revelations. It was found that many of the stores paid such small salaries that to live on them at all was an impossibility for even the most economical. It was an understood fact that each girl was expected to receive help from some "gentleman friend."

There must be something wrong in our whole system of living when girls are compelled to work for salaries insufficient for even the necessities and are taught to have tastes and desires for the beautiful which it is impossible to gratify on their meager salaries. A young girl goes to work in an office or store with a definite, if not expressed, understanding of what should be the proper relations of the sexes. After she has been at work a short time she notices that her companions are much better dressed than it is possible for her to be with the resources at her command. She notices that her friends have numerous invitations to theatres and dinners. She wonders if she is less attractive than they. After awhile she receives hints, more or less broad, from her male associates. Gradually it dawns upon her why the other girls are more attractive than she.

One who has not been thrown in close contact with the girls of this age cannot realize the extent of the immorality among them. Formerly it was considered that only boys sowed their wild oats. Now we find that many girls do so also. We hear very little about it except for the occasional case of one who has to suffer for her sins. Usually this one is one of the most innocent. Many of the girls of this generation are "wise." They think they know how to "keep out of trouble," and yet reap the rewards in the shape of a few dollars.

Girls cannot afford to take the great risks incident to leading an immoral life, aside from all moral reasons for not doing so. In the first place there is the danger of becoming pregnant. Think what that means! The majority of girls are led to take the first step by promises of marriage. Real life has proved these promises seldom are kept. The man "changes" his mind after the mis-step has been taken. He goes away and forgets, the girl is left to bear the consequences of their mutual sin. The men of the world like to take these girls out and enjoy themselves but when it comes to marriage--the man wants a different kind of a wife. There are three courses from which such an unfortunate girl may choose. One course is an abortion with all its attendant dangers, its risks to her life and the thoughts of having taken a life. Another is to brave the world, bear her child and keep it. It takes a great deal of courage to do this with our present social system. Often it is impossible, as the girl is unable to care for the child and at the same time support it and herself. She seldom finds very much encouragement in this course. Those who should be her friends and aid her to make the most of her life are now the ones who keep her down. They refuse to make it possible for her to earn an honest living and lead a moral life. The third course is to place herself under the care of a responsible physician, live in seclusion for the last few months of her pregnancy, then, after the birth of her baby, have it adopted. Considering everything, this often is the best course. From the child's standpoint, it is given a better start in life. It is much better to live as the adopted, but honored, child in a home than it is to have to bear the stigma of illegitimacy. As soon as the child enters school the latter will become known among its playmates and will be the subject of many cruel taunts. It is not fair to the innocent child to give it such a heritage. But think how the mothers must feel to have to give up their babies! That is the saddest part of the case. It is not fair that the girl should be punished the remainder of her life for one mis-step when the man goes absolutely free and without the sign of a stigma attached to him.

These cases of unfortunate girls are all too common. The rescue homes in the large cities are full, and often a large percentage of their occupants are from the country. Within the last week, I have received letters from four girls, similar to the one I shall read you. This letter is from a girl in Indiana who gives a rural delivery address. "In one of your articles in ---- you speak of homes where unfortunate girls are sheltered and taken care of and I should like to know if there is such a home in Indianapolis. If there is, will you kindly give me the street and number. I am in trouble and have nowhere to go, but knowing you to be a friend to unfortunate girls who met their misfortune through ignorance and with no desire to do wrong, I write you for advice." This, as well as numerous other letters, show that these things are just as prevalent in the country districts as in the cities.

So many girls do not realize how easy it is to "get into trouble." A short time ago I had a confinement case that was a little unusual; for the young woman, who was unmarried, had an unruptured hymen, which contained only one small opening barely large enough to insert a sound the size of a slate pencil. At the first consultation several months previous, when she had come to me on account of absence of menstruation for three months, the girl had insisted that there was no possibility of her being pregnant. Later she admitted that four months previously, just after she menstruated, she was out with a young man who was very insistent, that she did not consent, but in spite of her resistance there was a discharge thrown against the labia (external organs). At the time of this first examination she was about four months pregnant and had not supposed such a condition of affairs possible. Fortunately in this case there was an early marriage.

Another grave danger to the girl who indulges in immoral practices is the possibility of contracting one of the black plagues. You know what that would mean. If you recall the prevalence of these diseases you will see that the probabilities are that any girl indulging in immoral relations will sooner or later contract one of these diseases. Indeed she runs a big risk of contracting one at her first mis-step.

After one has taken the first mis-step it is very easy to take the next. One step often leads to another until the girl succumbs to a life of prostitution. A result of prostitution that is important is the unfitting for regular life. Whatever the effect of such a life may be upon a man, a girl cannot lead such a life with impunity. Many a girl tires of her immoral life and gladly would turn to something else but the difficulties in her way are numerous. One is her inability to obtain a position when it is known that she has led an immoral life. Another is that she finds the duties and regular hours incident to any position very irksome. The irregular life she has led has unfitted her for a regular life. There seems to have been a general disturbance of the whole nervous system, her will has become so weakened that it is very hard for her to have the will power necessary to keep from returning to the old life. This breaking of the will power also makes it difficult for her to keep her mind on her work. Then, too, she resents any supervision of her work. Of course, the longer the irregular life has continued the harder it is to break away from it.

Now, from another standpoint! No matter how dissipated a man may be he wants his bride to be pure. Nearly all girls expect to marry sometime, and so for the sake of the future--in order to keep the confidence of her husband as well as for the sake of not taking any risks that might prevent future motherhood, girls should not lead immoral lives.

CHAPTER XVIII

FLIRTATIONS AND THEIR RESULTS

The greater social freedom of the present generation without adequate preparation has resulted in an increasing tendency among young girls to make chance acquaintances and perhaps clandestine engagements. That these flirtations, entered into so innocently, may result in events that will be the cause of lifelong regret is seldom realized by a young girl. Yet very often such is the case!

One letter I received says, "I will give you a short outline of my life since last April when my troubles began, for which I blame my parents partly, because I was not allowed to have my friends at my home or go out with young men, as the other girls do, with my parents' knowledge of it and because I was kept ignorant of the things I think every girl should know. I was nineteen last March. The men say I am the kind that looks good to men, that they cannot resist. As to this I do not know, but I do know that I always attract their attentions and I am sorry that I do. And yet I crave them. I have for years and I am lonesome without them. I want their friendship and company. I do not know why it is but I am more satisfied with the boys than the girls. Last April a young man, somewhere in the thirties, I think, though he looked much younger, came to our little country town. He was handsome, well educated, finely dressed and always seemed to have plenty of money. I was very unhappy about this time over my troubles at home and because my boy friend, who always had been a friend through all, had for some cause unknown to me stopped writing to me. So I met the young man first in company with friends a couple of times, then he wished to make an appointment to meet me alone and, through the kindness of my friends, I met him out at night several times. On the third night before I half realized what I was doing I had let him ruin me. I had never been told that this was wrong and yet I seemed to know that it was. It worried me, but there was no one I could go to for advice and my friend said that since what was done already could never be undone I might as well keep it up, etc. Having no advice but his, I followed it and for several weeks met him out any and every where and time I could. I knew of the trouble that might come from these meetings and asked my friend about it but he said that everything was all right, that he would tend to that and that nothing would happen. But it did happen. He was going away in a few days and gave me some medicine to take, telling me I was only held back on account of it being the first time. But I didn't believe him and went to a married lady whom I had known but a short time but whom I thought I could trust and who would help me. She invited my friend and me there one evening and talked the matter over with us or rather with him. He stayed over and helped me out of my trouble. But my health has never been the same since. Now, what I want to ask you is this, do you think it would be right for me to marry any man, with him thinking that I am good or innocent? Do men expect that of the women they marry? But I do not wish to marry if I can help it, but I must do something. I will go crazy if I stay here at home from worrying over what I have done and for fear my parents will find it out. What I wish to do is to go away to work, but I have no one to go to and am afraid I cannot resist the temptations that they say come to every working girl. I have given in twice since my trouble, both times shortly afterwards. The first because I could not help it and the second because I was afraid of being told on, he having been told by the first man. But when I found out I could not resist the teasing I quit going out and it has been months since I have been out with a man and I am trying to lead a decent life but it is hard and at times it seems that I must give in. Now, please write and tell me just exactly what you think of my case. Has my whole life been ruined by this man?"

Unless this girl will "play soldier" and "right about face" she is in danger of landing in a house of ill-fame. How common is her story! Girls do not realize what are the possible results that may follow an innocent flirtation. Young girls are not posted and they do not know men. They do not realize the pressure that will be brought to bear upon them. Many young girls grow to womanhood without any idea of the relations of the sexes. To them, love is devoid of ideas of sex, practically the same as their love for a brother or sister. It is not until they are thrown alone in the company of some older man that they suddenly awaken to a realization of what it all means.

The girls who like to be petted, to be kissed and hugged can see no harm in that and do not realize what a sleeping force may be aroused. The man, when he finds a girl will allow these attentions, thinks that she knows what they may lead to and naturally assumes that she is willing, but only wishes to be coaxed. It is a clear case of misunderstanding on both sides. But that does not make the consequences any less harmful.

Girls do not realize what kind of an impression they make upon men by their clothes, actions, etc. An eminent lawyer said to me recently, "Why do you not tell girls what real men think of them when they appear on the streets with painted faces, peek-a-boo waists and thin, silk hose worn with shoes more appropriate for the ball-room? If girls imitate the demi-monde in their dress they must expect to be treated accordingly." There is in every girl's nature a desire to appear attractive in the eyes of those of the opposite sex and this desire leads them to extremes of dressing. These extremes of dressing naturally attract the attention of men, and the girls feel flattered and continue in their course, not realizing what impression the men really get. Then, when the man makes the advances that her manner of dressing has led him to believe he can make, she feels insulted and resentful.

The fault lies in the fact that the girl has not been properly educated and has received exaggerated and entirely wrong ideas of life.

CHAPTER XIX

WHITE SLAVERY

During the past few years the public has been much interested in the prosecution of the white slave investigation. Every adult person had a more or less definite idea that there were in existence immoral houses. But the majority of women had no idea that their existence should be of any especial interest to them.

The Hon. Edwin Sims, U. S. District Attorney, Chicago, says: "There are some things so far removed from the lives of normal, decent people as to be simply unbelievable by them. The 'white slave' trade of to-day is one of these incredible things. The calmest, simplest statements of its facts are almost beyond the comprehension of belief of men and women who are mercifully spared from contact with the dark and hideous secrets of the 'under-world' of the big cities.

"Naturally, wisely, every parent who reads this statement will at once raise the question: 'What excuse is there for the open discussion of such a revolting condition of things? What good is there to be served by flaunting so dark and disgusting a subject before the family circle?' Only one--and that is a reason and not an excuse! The recent examination of more than two hundred 'white slaves' by the office of the U. S. District Attorney at Chicago has brought to light the fact that literally thousands of innocent girls from the country districts are every year entrapped into a life of hopeless slavery and degradation because parents in the country do not understand conditions as they exist and how to protect their daughters from the 'white slave' traders who have reduced the art of ruining young girls to a national and international system. I sincerely believe that nine-tenths of the parents of these thousands of girls who are every year snatched from lives of decency and comparative peace and dragged under the slime of an existence in the 'white slave world' have no idea that there is really a trade in the ruin of girls as much as there is a trade in cattle or sheep or other products of the farm.

"I have no disposition to add a single word to what will open the eyes of parents to the fact that white slavery is an existing condition--a system of girl hunting that is national and international in its scope, that it literally consumes thousands of girls--clean, innocent girls--every year; that it is operated with a cruelty, a barbarism that gives a new meaning to the word fiend; that it is an imminent peril to every girl in the country who has a desire to get into the city and taste its excitement and pleasures."

One of the worst obstacles to be overcome in the work of protecting innocent girls and restoring to useful lives those who have been betrayed, is the blind incredulity on the part of a large percentage of the public. There are thousands of women all over the country who know as little about what is going on in the world as do so many children. They are wonderfully ignorant of the terrible conditions that are in existence all around them. Of course their blindness to these awful conditions makes them more peaceful and contented for the time being than they possibly could be if they realized the temptations and perils that are lying in wait for their daughters and the daughters of their friends. But this peace is not permanent and every year thousands of mothers are rudely awakened from their sleep of peace to find that while they were asleep to the perils of the world their daughters have been drawn into the whirlpool. The awakening of such parents comes too late usually to do any good. The recent agitation along this line has caused many a mother to exclaim, "How terrible; I did not dream that such a condition of affairs could exist in this country."

If you possessed a rare jewel and knew you were surrounded by those who would try to obtain possession of that jewel you would not entrust it to a blind or a deaf watchman or one so ignorant of the wiles of the robbers that he would trustingly allow it to pass into their possession. There is nothing in the world so priceless to the father and mother as the virtue and happiness of their daughter. And yet there are thousands of parents who have been entrusted with the care of a daughter who are trying to discharge that trust with their eyes blinded and their ears closed. They insist upon keeping the childish belief that there is no real danger threatening their daughter. These parents do not live in the world. They fold their hands and raise their eyes towards heaven and cry, "Peace! Peace!" and are unable to see the enemy slipping upon their daughter to drag her down to a life of shame.

In this age no young girl is beyond temptation. She needs all the protection possible, and in order to protect her the parents must be awake to the dangers and provided with the best means of protection. One of the things hardest to make honest and trusting parents believe is that there can be people in the world who make it their business to lead girls into a life of shame. But such is the case whether we believe it or not. The men and women who ply this trade lay their plans more carefully and employ more artifices than can be conceived of by the ordinary parent. The wonder is that not more are caught in the net.

Another fact which the public finds it hard to believe is that the girls who are lured into the life of shame find it impossible to escape from such a life, that they are prisoners and slaves in every sense of the word.

The artifices employed by these slave-dealers to obtain their victims are many and frequently are so adroitly formulated as to blind not only the victim but her parents as well.

One common trick of these slave procurers is the promise of a good position. Many a girl has gone to the cities thinking she had obtained a definite and desirable position. Perhaps she was to be met at the station by the person who obtained the position for her. Too late she finds her position is in a house of ill-fame. So common has this trick become that in every large city there are organizations of social workers who offer through the churches to look up the desirability of any position which has been obtained by a girl so that should it prove to be a lure of the destroyer she could be warned before it was too late.

Another favorite device of the white slaver for landing victims is the runaway marriage trick. The alleged summer resorts and excursion centers which are so widely advertised as Gretna Greens and as places where the usual legal and official formalities preliminary to respectable marriage are reduced to the minimum are star recruiting stations for the white slave traffic. So common is this trick that a wise mother would refuse to allow her daughter to visit one of these places or to go on one of the pleasure excursions unless accompanied by some older member of the family. Also, every mother should teach her daughter that any man who proposed such a marriage was to be looked upon with suspicion, and should not be trusted for an instant.

Then there is the restaurant trick. The girl is induced to go to what she thinks is a restaurant and then perhaps is taken into a private room only to find that this room leads to her prison. Girls cannot be too suspicious of going to unknown places with comparative strangers--either men or women.

The moving picture shows furnish to these slavers another opportunity of misleading girls. These shows naturally attract children and very young girls. Evidence has been procured which proves that many girls owe their ruin to frequenting them. As an instance of this, three girls met as many young men at a moving picture show and at the end of the performance were induced to leave the theater by a side door which was found to open into an adjoining building and all passed the night together.

The massage parlors and manicure parlors upon investigation proved to have been used as a bait for these vile procurers. Many of these places were found to be not equipped for their legitimate work but to be nothing more than disorderly houses.

The investigations of the United States courts have resulted in the imprisonment of many of these panders but there are many more still unconvicted and the danger to young girls is ever present. The parents cannot be too watchful in their protection, and to be watchful they must be cognizant of the dangers and of the methods in use. The daughters must be so educated that they are prepared to cope with the enemy. Remember, as Browning says, "Ignorance is not innocence, but sin."

CHAPTER XX

THE NEED OF EARLY INSTRUCTION OF BOYS

I have made so emphatic the necessity of early and proper instruction of girls and I have shown you that so much of the disease and unhappiness in the world is due to this lack of instruction that I do not believe any of your daughters ever will say, "Why was I not told these things before it was too late?" But you women will have sons as well as daughters and you are just as responsible for their future happiness as you are for that of your daughters. Besides the future happiness of another woman's daughter depends in a large measure upon the health of your son. The boys need instruction as much if not more than do the girls; at any rate they need it earlier than the girls do, because boys talk more freely than girls and boys acquire their first impressions of these subjects much earlier than girls.

No boy ever willfully contracted a disease that would produce so much future misery as that resulting from one of the venereal diseases. You remember I made the remark that the large percentage of men contracted these diseases before their twentieth year, before they had any adequate knowledge of the possible consequences. If boys were warned there would be no more of this innocent acquisition of disease. Many a man has had cause to regret all his life a few moments of thoughtless dissipation. Even though a boy has acquired one of these diseases that is no reason why he should suffer from it the remainder of his life any more than that he constantly should suffer from an attack of smallpox. One difference at the present time is that the smallpox patient receives the most scientific treatment procurable, but the victim of one of these plagues is neglected. Boys are told these diseases are no worse than a cold and so do not realize the necessity for prompt and adequate treatment. The ordinary boy treats himself, following the advice of some of his friends or some incompetent person. He has a feeling of shame which prevents him from going to the family physician, who would give him honest advice. If he goes to any physician he usually goes to some advertising physician who claims to be a "men specialist." The main speciality of these men is obtaining money from their ignorant dupes. Their advertisements would make nearly every man in the world think he were suffering from some grave disease. The young boy, at an impressionable age, is a ready victim to their lures. He is treated for a real or an imaginary disease until his money is all gone, then he is discharged.

Let me read you a letter I received from a young boy which will illustrate my meaning: "I read your article 'A Father's Duty to His Son,' in the ---- and take the liberty of writing to you. My father died when I was but nine years old, so

I was left to my own resources, the result being I am now a nervous wreck at the age of nineteen. I have doctored for nervous debility with four doctors for over a year and a half. The result, they got every cent out of me but did not help me a particle. If my mother ever found it out, it would worry her to death, as she has hopes in me, fool that I was. My condition, I am always nervous when in company, expecting somebody to accuse me any minute. My eyes always are blurred and my hands shake as if I were an old man. I have night losses, which bother me more than anything and if they stopped I know I could fight my way back to health. If you could possibly give me some recipe or advice it would be greatly appreciated. Nobody but one in this condition can imagine the strain on the mind and body. Although I feel well when alone, though awfully weak, I am a nervous wreck when in the presence of others. I have written to you because your article seems to tell facts which I know to be true."

Now, if you will pardon me I will quote a portion of my reply: "Evidently you have been the victim of unscrupulous doctors. Unfortunately there are a number. They usually advertise themselves as specialists in diseases of men. A reliable physician does not advertise. If you had gone to a trustworthy family physician in the first place you would have been saved much worry, and incidentally considerable money.

"The chief advice you need is to stop worrying. The night losses you mention are a natural condition. They occur with nearly every normal man who is living a continent life. Even if they occur two or three times a week they do not indicate any diseased condition. The more you worry and think about such things the more often they will occur. I do not know what your occupation is, but if it is indoor work you must plan to take a great deal of outdoor exercise every day. If you could go out in the country for awhile and do hard outdoor work it would be the best thing for you. Eat only plain, easily digested food, but eat plenty. Do not use any condiments nor stimulants. Sleep on a hard bed with plenty of fresh air in the room. Bathe the external genitals with cold water night and morning.... The fact that you have abused yourself in the past need not prevent you from being a perfectly healthy person now if you are not continuing the practice."

Every boy desires to be a man but does not quite understand the meaning of the word. He dislikes to be called a "greeny" or anything that suggests that he is young and inexperienced. Often he pretends to know things he does not. Nearly every boy, at an early age, is thrown in contact with low-minded persons who think it amusing to persuade the youth to prove he knows indecent things. He thinks it a test of manhood to be acquainted with various vices and so in order to prove his knowledge is led into various indiscretions, which result in the contraction of vile habits or of loathsome diseases.

If a boy at an early age were given the true idea of the meaning of being a man or of manhood we would have fewer physical wrecks and incompetent individuals.

CHAPTER XXI

WHY BOYS GO ASTRAY

"What can a boy do, and where can a boy stay, If he is always told to get out of the way? He cannot sit here, and he must not stand there, The cushions that cover that fine rocking chair Were put there, of course, to be seen and admired; A boy has no business to ever be tired. The beautiful roses and flowers that bloom On the floor of the darkened and delicate room Are made not to walk on--at least, not by boys; The house is no place, anyway, for their noise, Yet boys must walk somewhere, and what if their feet, Sent out of their houses, sent into the street, Should step round the corner and pause at the door Where other boys' feet have paused often before; Should pass the gateway of glittering light, Where jokes that are merry and songs that are bright Ring out a warm welcome with flattering voice, And temptingly say, 'Here's a place for the boys.'

"Ah, what if they should? What if your boy or mine Should cross o'er the threshold which marks out the line 'Twixt virtue and vice, 'twixt pureness and sin, And leave all his innocent boyhood within? Oh, what if they should, because you and I While the days and the months and the years hurry by, Are too busy with cares and with life's fleeting joys To make round our hearthstone a place for the boys? There's a place for the boys. They'll find it somewhere; And if our own homes are too daintily fair For the touch of their fingers, the tread of their feet, They'll find it, and find it, alas, in the street, 'Mid the gilding of sin and the glitter of vice; And with heartaches and longings we pay a dear price For the getting of gain that our lifetime employs, If we fail to provide a good place for the boys."

This little poem, published anonymously in a country newspaper, seems to me to tell the story of why boys go astray. They are not understood at home and so naturally go where someone seems to understand and want them.

In a great many homes the boy's room is a very unattractive place, merely a place in which to sleep. He is not allowed in the "parlor." He always seems to be in the way. No one seems to take any interest in the things that are closest to his heart. It is only natural that he should gradually drift to the saloon, the billiard room, the questionable houses, because he is made to feel that he is welcome there. Indeed his tastes and desires are consulted there.

A boy always is interested in sex problems. The vulgar delight in feeding his fancy, in giving him exaggerated ideas of these much abused subjects. He is lead on from one step to another. Often many of the things he does are performed in a spirit of bravado, simply because he does not wish to appear "green."

From one of the reliable magazines comes this information: "Forty-one families--'nice families,' as we call them--were last May thrown into consternation and humiliation by being privately notified by the head master of a boys' school that their boys would not be re 雄 tered for another term at his school. 'A fearful condition of immorality,' wrote the head master, 'has been unearthed at the school, and in order to set an example to the rest of the boys, every boy concerned will be denied re 雄 trance to this school.'

"The 'fearful condition of immorality' discovered in the school was, as the head master privately explained, traceable, as it generally is, 'to one boy, the son of a family of unquestioned standing in its community,' and he has involved the other boys.

"The boy in question was not a vicious lad: on the contrary, he was a boy possessed of more than ordinary good characteristics. When he was brought up before the head master and the full result of his baneful influence was explained to him the boy was panic stricken.

"'Didn't you realize what you were doing?' asked the head master.

"'No,' replied the boy, who was nineteen and really a young man: 'I knew it was wrong, yes, but I didn't realize how wrong. As a matter of fact,' said the boy, 'I didn't know what I was doing, and how I was getting the boys into a thing that I now see is more serious than I had any idea of.'

"'Didn't your father and mother ever explain these things to you?' asked the head master.

"'Not a word,' answered the boy, and then as a grim look came on his face he said: 'God! I wish they had!'

"A pleasant realization must it be to the parents of this boy as they read this sentence in the head master's letter to the father of this boy:

"'I cannot but feel that your criminal negligence in the most vital duty that can come to a parent is the direct cause in this twofold calamity: first, of the downfall of your own son; and second, of the downfall of each of the other forty boys, and of the humiliation in which they and their parents find themselves. These are hard words to say to you, but they are true, and I say them not alone as the head master of this school, but also as one father to another, and as one man to another.'"

In the growing youth's mind there arise many questions that he would like to talk over with his father, but he feels diffident about asking him. Too often the boy grows up and goes away to college without ever talking with his father about manhood. In all matters concerning his business relations and success, the boy has received careful instruction. He has not been left to work out those problems by himself but is given the benefit of the experiences of those who have trodden the road before. But in this matter so vital to his whole life, he has been left to clear his own path through the woods. With no guide and bewildered with the new ideas and experiences that crowd upon him, is it any wonder he loses his way, wanders off the straight path, falls ofttimes into some bog that perhaps was hidden from his sight by surrounding flowers and to which he has been lured by siren music?

The father's duty to his son is plain--and must not be neglected. In some cases the mother must attend to this duty and for the future welfare of her son she must see that he receives adequate instruction.

CHAPTER XXII

HOW SHALL THE CHILD BE TOLD?

Every mother and every father realizes that there are certain things incident to reproduction that must be learned by the child at an early age. They realize, too, that it is preferable that this information should be imparted by the parents. But, on account of their own lack of instruction, they find two problems confronting them. How and when shall I tell my child are the questions uppermost in many parents' minds.

The answer to the first question must depend upon the individual case. At a certain age a baby expresses a desire for something to bite. Before that time we make no effort to force him to bite. Later he finds he can help himself from one position to another by creeping. Then in a few months he discovers he is able to use his feet and tries to walk. We do not try to force any of these new ideas upon him but simply wait patiently until he expresses a desire to acquire some new knowledge, then we aid him and guide his efforts.

There comes a time in the life of every child when he awakens to knowledge of reproduction. Then is the time to give the information. Some children commence to inquire as early as three years. At such an early age it is not necessary to go into details, as a very little information suffices to satisfy the child.

Just how to tell the truths necessary must vary with the age of the child. It is important to remember to be truthful to the child. When a mother tells the child that the stork or the doctor brings the baby, she sets a seal upon evasion. Some day he will learn that his mother has deceived him and that behind her instruction lies an element of secrecy, and secrecy with its companion curiosity is the cause of much unrest in after life. The child gathers the idea that there must be something shameful connected with the birth of a child or his mother would not be ashamed to tell him the truth.

Secondly, the child must be told scientifically that this knowledge may form a basis for later studies in biology. He can be taught in a simple manner that all nature comes from a seed; that the mother makes a tiny nest for the seed and that with all seeds it is necessary for their growth that the father gives them some pollen.

Until these subjects are put before children and young people with some degree of intelligence and sympathetic handling, it cannot be expected that anything but the utmost confusion in mind and in morals should reign in matters of sex. It seems incredible that our thoughts could be so unclean that we find it impossible to give to our children the information they need on these most sacred subjects, but instead we allow them to obtain their information whenever and wherever they can and in the most unclean manner. A child at the age of puberty is capable of the most sensitive, affectional and serene appreciation of what sex means and can absorb the teachings if properly given without any shock to his sense of the fitness of things. Indeed whenever these subjects are taught to the child correctly they induce a feeling of reverence for the mother that could not otherwise be obtained. A little child when told that she grew in a nest in mother's body right underneath mother's heart at once becomes filled with a great love and wonder for that mother. Then later to teach the relation of fatherhood and how the love of parents for each other and their desire to have a child of their very own was the cause of that child's existence--these things seem so natural to the child mind that has not been polluted with vulgar ideas that they excite in him no sense of unfitness, only a deep gratitude and a kind of tender wonderment.

The great point to remember in teaching these things to children is to satisfy their present question and leave the understanding that mother (or father) always stands ready and willing to explain any problems that are bothering the child.

So many girls have told me that when they were between six and fourteen years of age they had heard some things about the land where the babies grow and immediately went to their mothers and inquired as to the truth of what they had heard. The invariable answer received was, "Little girls must not talk about such things." That silenced the child and the mother heaved a sigh of relief that the question had passed off so smoothly and easily. That little sentence has been the cause of innumerable mistakes and misery. That little sentence marked the beginning of the failure of the child to confide in her mother, the child never again would broach the subject to her mother. However, that did not mean that the child would not receive the information requested; for, as a rule, the girls who told of this incidence also remarked that they had received the information very soon from some older girl and frequently in a vulgar manner. If a mother wishes to retain the confidence of her daughter, if a father wishes to retain the confidence of his son they both must keep a keen lookout for the first questions and be prepared to answer them at the time.

Later on the special sexual needs of the boy or the girl can be explained, the necessity of cleanliness and the danger of self-abuse. The need of self-control and the possibility of deflecting physical desire to other channels and the great gain resulting; all these things the youth of either sex are capable of understanding and appreciating, and the knowledge given early will prevent many physical and moral wrecks.

It is the duty of fathers and mothers to prepare themselves on these subjects so as to have the answer ready when the child first inquires. There is no excuse for not doing so, for educators all over the country stand ready to help any parents who call upon them. It is possible for every community to obtain the services of a lecturer or teacher who will instruct the parents. The individual can obtain books which explain all these things simply and plainly. There is no excuse for ignorance.

CHAPTER XXIII

WOMEN IN BUSINESS

If all homes were ideal and all men likewise, there would be no question of woman suffrage or woman in business. But this is not an ideal world; all women who have kept their places and stayed at home, kept house and taken care of their children have not led ideal lives. In too many instances the home woman, the little wren, has been deserted for the gay song-bird. The necessities of life have forced other women into the business world--women whose preference would be for the ideal, quiet home life. One must not think that because a woman is leading a public life that she prefers it, that she has no desire for a home and little ones. Often her choice has been the lesser of two evils,--more to be desired than a life, married, but loveless; one in which she must slave from morn till eve and then receive as recompense curses and fault-finding.

The woman who refuses to so demean the married life as to enter into such a marriage, preferring instead the busy life of a bachelor maid, is to be admired rather than condemned. That she makes a success of her business life tends to show what some man has missed by not proving himself worthy to be her husband.

We hear so much about woman entering into business--just as though she had not always been in business. Stop and think about our ancestors on the farms. The woman shared the work equally with the man. He attended to the heavier work, while she attended to that which required less physical strength but more attention to details. The products of her industry often brought as much ready cash as that derived from the sale of the larger products of the farm. Many families depended for the yearly supply of clothes and luxuries on the money thus obtained from the sale of butter, eggs and chickens. In olden days, too, many a woman derived an income from the sale of home-made rugs and counterpanes.

Just how men have conceived the idea that it is only the modern woman who is a money earner, I cannot understand, nor can I understand how some men expect women to be happy in idleness. The most unhappy women in the world are the women who have a great deal of leisure time. Many a man objects to his wife taking up any outside work even though it would not interfere with her household duties. This usually is due to false pride on his part. He is afraid of what others will say; afraid his friends will think he is not capable of supporting his wife. Some of these men forget to take into account the possibility that an accident or illness may take him away, business failures may sweep away his accumulations and then his wife must face the necessity of earning her living. Alas, how seldom is she prepared to do this! If, during the leisure time of her protected life, she had been perfecting herself in some branch of industry, her future would be easily solved.

A woman can devote several hours a day to outside affairs and still not neglect her home duties. Home-making does not necessarily mean that the woman herself must do the washing, ironing, cooking, baking or sewing. She must see that these are performed properly but the actual work may all be done by others. A business man does not attempt to do all the work of the office himself. He employs a bookkeeper, a clerk and a stenographer to attend to the details while he directs. It is the same way with a home, a woman may employ others to do the physical labor while she directs.

Then as to the married woman earning money. Let me give you an illustration. A woman has spent the early part of her life perfecting herself in some branch of work, for instance, book cover designing. She marries a man in moderate circumstances and does not feel that she can afford to be idle and employ someone else to do her house work. She is a slenderly built woman and it would be a great tax on her strength to perform all the household duties--for some parts of housekeeping require such hard physical labor that even many men would not care to attempt them. It certainly would seem a very reasonable thing for this woman to devote several hours a day to book cover designing and use the money so earned to employ a strong woman to do the heavy housework. This arrangement would be better for all concerned; first, the woman would be happier and more contented; next, the man would enjoy his home more, for any man certainly would rather come home and find his wife contented and happy and with leisure time to devote to him, than to come home and find her all tired out, and consequently cross, with the housework so unfinished she must devote her evening to some household task.

If circumstances have given a woman home and children, they always must come first, but this does not mean the woman must do housework if conditions permit the employment of somebody to do it. She must do the work for which she is best fitted both by nature and by training.

In whatever occupation a woman is engaged she should endeavor to make a success of that work, to do it a little better than anyone else could; for in every field of endeavor there is joy and reward for always being and doing one's best. The great secret of success is concentration. Too many women waste their energies thinking and talking about the things they would like to do. Every time you talk about the thing you would like to do you waste just that much energy and make your goal less possible of achievement. That which seems difficult before is usually found easy to accomplish, once undertaken. If you wish to accomplish anything hold the thought in your mind and concentrate all your powers in that direction. Do not scatter your energies like chaff to be blown hither and thither.

CHAPTER XXIV

NERVOUSNESS--A LACK OF CONTROL

How often do we meet women who complain of being nervous. What they really mean is that they have not control of their nerves but let them run away. A woman may be of a nervous temperament and yet have such good control of her nerves that she never complains of being nervous. This lack of nerve control manifests itself in various ways. Sometimes it only is a tendency to cry at trivial things or an inclination to despondency--to have "the blues," or to worry over real or fancied slights. Many women waste so much time thinking over things that are past and gone. A visit with a friend loses its joy in the afterthought, for this victim of the nerves lives over again every moment of the visit. She recalls everything that has been said and wonders if a different meaning were meant. Things that were said as a joke and originally taken that way now are brought up for criticism and pondered over until the woman convinces herself of the presence of a hidden meaning. She is not satisfied until she has bent and shapen the original thoughtless sentence into an ugly sting.

These nervous women are the ones who continually are tormented with the demon of jealousy. If one of them should suddenly meet her husband on the street walking with another woman, what a curtain lecture he would receive that evening; or if not that, he finds his wife wearing the air of one who considers herself much abused. The real facts of the case may be that her husband met the other woman quite accidentally and, as they were going in the same direction, he could not avoid walking with her without being positively rude. In this age men must, of necessity, have business transactions with women. It is a common occurrence for two men to lunch together in order to have a chance to talk over some important business without fear of interruption. There is no reason why a man and woman might not do the same, and yet how impossible it would be to convince the jealous woman that this was the case. To be jealous is to acknowledge the superior charms of the other woman. "If I cannot hold you against all women, then I do not want you." If you think some other woman is attracting your husband, wake up and beat her at her own game. Do not sit idly in the corner and complain. You only are making yourself miserable and not trying to right the wrong.

A woman who is nervous usually does not realize what is the cause of her condition. When excitable and irritable and suffering from a nervous headache, she takes various remedies to deaden the symptoms, instead of looking the matter squarely in the face and going after the cause.

Many women need a hobby to take up their spare time and to occupy their minds. If their minds are occupied and their bodies kept in good condition by proper care, they soon will gain control of their nerves. If you find yourself getting nervous, make up your mind to overcome it by filling your life so full of work and play that you will have no time to give way to the nerves. When you feel an attack coming on, get busy and "work it off."

There is a class of women who possess comfortable homes, with a maid to do the work, whose home duties are not confining and who find themselves with a great deal of extra time on their hands. To these women the days are long and they endeavor to pass away the time by doing nerve racking fancy work or by "fussing" around the house. They are not happy and contented, chiefly because their minds are being neglected--are growing up to weeds like a neglected garden. For such a woman club work is a boon. She should take up some especial kind of work, and devote several hours a day to the study of it. At first this will be hard, for a mind that has fallen into lazy ways is not easily aroused to continual effort, the deeply rooted weeds are not easily destroyed.

Many half contented women realize this need of mental food but hesitate. As one woman said, "Why, my husband would leave me if I started to work!"

Some men take a peculiar attitude towards women. They would like to treat them as a woman treats her pet dog. The dog is provided with a comfortable home, plenty of food, someone to bathe it and carry it around. The dog is contented with this. It loves to sleep and eat the livelong day; it comes when its mistress calls, and goes when she is tired of it. Unfortunately, perhaps, all women cannot be contented with such a life. The woman was given a brain which refuses to be dormant. If it is not required to be used in a useful way, it occupies itself with bad thoughts--it worries and becomes fault finding or gossiping.

No woman should allow her mind to grow up to such weeds. If the circumstances of her position, her education or her environment seem to make it unwise that she take up any work that would bring a monetary reward, she easily can find some charitable work that needs all the energies she can devote to it. If such a woman would take up some special branch of philanthropic work she would be amply rewarded, not only by the consciousness of the good she had done, but by the improvement in her own health and happiness.

There is another phase to this lack of nerve control shown in a nervous tension, an inability to relax and enjoy life. Some people go through the day on such a nervous tension that they are unable to take cognizance of their surroundings. Eventually this tension will manifest itself in some disorder, as headache, nervous indigestion or complete nervous prostration. In the latter case the nerves have been so abused, so strained that at last they are worn out. A rest is imperative!

A woman who, if she has a few spare moments, can lie down and relax absolutely, perhaps even drop to sleep, has a better chance to stand the stress and strain of business or of housekeeping than the one who finds it impossible to do so. Try making it a point to lie down for two or three minutes several times a day; lie flat on your back and relax every muscle; put every worry or ugly thought out of your mind by thinking some pleasant but soothing sentence as, "I am glad I can rest. I will be happy when I arise." You will be surprised at the effect these few moments a day will produce upon your health and happiness.

Plenty of sleep is imperative for these women and yet so many of them neglect this great restorer of the nervous system. Frequently these women complain of an inability to go to sleep easily, and spend long hours of the night lying awake and entertaining worry thoughts. This symptom of disordered nerves should not be neglected. A warm bath before retiring, followed by a gentle massage, especially along the spine, will, by relaxing the nerves and muscles, produce very good results. A hot foot-bath, by drawing the blood away from the brain, often will be beneficial. A glass of hot milk or cocoa taken just before retiring may have the same effect. If the sleeplessness is a result of indigestion a plain diet will relieve. Sleeping upon a hard bed without a pillow sometimes produces the desired effect. Always have plenty of fresh air in the room. Keep the mind free from the cares of the day. If they will intrude crowd them out by repeating some soothing sentence as: "There is no reason why I should not sleep, therefore, I shall sleep. My body is relaxed, my mind is at peace, sleep is coming, I am getting sleepy, I am about to sleep." Never take any sleeping powders except upon the advice of a physician, for the majority of these sleeping powders contain some harmful drug, as morphine, codeine, phenacetin or acetanilid. The latter especially is very depressing to the heart and serves to weaken the nervous system. In fact many deaths may be laid at the door of these drugs. Treatments to tone up the nervous system and to improve the circulation often are indicated in these cases of "nerves." Control your nerves, do not let them control you!

CHAPTER XXV

A WOMAN IS AS YOUNG AS SHE WANTS TO BE

Have you ever thought why it is that some women are as young at forty as others are at twenty-four? And I mean young not frivolous! It is every woman's duty to keep young as long as possible, but, unfortunately, she does not always know the best way to live up to that duty. Keeping young means keeping your body in a perfectly healthy condition and your mind in harmony. With attention to certain laws a woman can detract ten years from her age. She can do this by treating herself as a friend and not as a slave. Take ten minutes and think how you could improve yourself by a little effort. Perhaps some of these suggestions will help you.

Everyone needs exercise. Just what sort depends upon the occupation of the individual. A woman doing housework exercises most of her muscles during the day, and if she makes pleasure, and not drudgery out of her work, this exercise is very beneficial. It is a pleasure to be able to accomplish so much, but the housework is not sufficient exercise. This woman needs exercise for her mind and for her beauty-loving soul. In her spare time she should lie under the trees and enjoy nature or a good book, or she should go to some gathering where she will meet those who will refresh her intellectually. Keep the mind open to all the impressions of nature. Love the open air. Fresh air is not a fad, it is a necessity if one would keep young. Occasionally read a book of travel or a biography of some well-known person. Keep mentally alert. An intellectual back number adds years to her seeming age. Nothing makes for youth as a young mind, save perhaps a young heart.

If a woman wishes to retain her attractiveness and not grow dull and uninteresting, she must be interested in the outside world. Make it a point to go somewhere every day. If you cannot do anything else, put the baby in the cart and walk a few blocks. Do not say you are too busy. It is necessary for your health and you will find a few minutes' outing will give you renewed energies and help you to see the silver lining. If possible go to social affairs where you meet people. Invite others to your home but do not tire yourself entertaining them. People who are boarding enjoy a simple home-cooked meal. It is the "homey" air they enjoy and not elaborate decorations or menu.

A woman in an office needs different exercise. She needs to do something that will stretch and strengthen the tired muscles. She also needs plenty of fresh air. A brisk walk is one of the best exercises for her. Walk part of the way to the office, if possible, and keep your eyes open for interesting things you pass. Use your imagination in guessing the life story of those you meet. Forget yourself by becoming interested in others, and you will be surprised at the effect upon your outlook on life. It is not work that makes the business girl grow old and careworn as much as it is her inability to forget her work during her play or rest time. A business man takes an occasional day off and goes hunting or fishing, but the business girl seldom can afford the little trips that would serve to break the monotony of work. But every day brings its opportunities for little pleasures that are available. Remember it is the small things of life that make up its enjoyment. Once in a while at noon go to some especially nice lunch room where you will see well dressed women, where the service is faultless and every mouthful and every moment enjoyable. You will come away filled with such a sense of well-being that you will be able to accomplish twice as much in the way of work. Many business girls do not entertain themselves well enough. They become so imbued with the spirit of economy that they deny themselves the little pleasures that would make life enjoyable. This reacts upon their work and ability. These people who continually stint themselves never achieve great success. They repress themselves so much that they quell all their best impulses. They never expand.

Learn self-control. Anger is a rapid wrinkle bringer. The energy that is wasted in useless worry and tirade against circumstances might be conserved and diverted into other channels that would bring you abundant reward, financially as well as in other ways. Avoid worry, hurry and getting flustered. Plan your work in the morning, then take the little interruptions coolly and quietly. You will not be half so tired at the end of the day as you would be otherwise. Be temperate. Moderation does not refer only to the stomach. Overdoing in any way makes for premature age.

Do not let yourself get sluggish and indifferent. Here is where the benefits of massage, physical culture and a vital interest in life come in. Youth is happiness! If you would be young, radiate happiness. Talk happiness not ill-health. One certain symptom of advancing age is the desire to talk about ill-health. Discussing operations you have undergone or sickness you have experienced always attracts attention to your age. Children seldom talk about ill-health. An illness once conquered is forgotten. Another thing, do not whine. The American women are noted for their unpleasant voices, which often are too high pitched, showing lack of control. Cultivate a low, well-modulated voice. Recently I met a young woman who had a deformed body and a plain face, but I immediately was attracted to her because she had the most beautiful speaking voice it ever was my privilege to hear.

As we age in years we are liable to grow careless in our dress, to select colors and styles that are not very becoming; we do not take as much pains with our hair, our nails or our shoes as we should. We have allowed age to manifest itself in the lack of care of the little things.

Finally, if your work does not bring you happiness, you are in the wrong place and the sooner you find the right place the better for you. It is impossible to take a race horse and expect to make him a good plow horse. We only would spoil the one without succeeding in obtaining the other. There is a right place for everyone and each one is adapted to certain things and in order to accomplish the most we must "find ourselves."